YOGA
Midlife Pain Relief Secrets

Discover Ancient Yoga Poses and Meditation
Techniques To Create A Holistic Mind-Body
Medicine Routine, Relieve Stress and
Achieve Pain Relief
…Even For Yoga Beginners!

by CATHERINE MAZUR

Interior and Cover Design by:
Rory Carruthers
www.RoryCarruthers.com

For more information about Catherine Mazur or to book her for your next event or media interview please visit: www.CatherineMazurYoga.com

Table of Contents

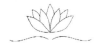

Preface

This book is a departure from traditional yoga. In it, I take liberty with the teachings of classical yoga, as well as modern day yoga practices. Drawing from my own experiences and the experiences of my students as we practice yoga, I will weave together current thought with ancient tradition. I'll present leading edge ideas from what we have learned about behavior and its correlation to the brain in order to give you the best of both worlds. From centuries old traditions to the latest in neuroscience and chemistry, we explore it all, using yogic principles as our jumping off point.

Steadily and unpredictably, the world changes. We are continually evolving individually and collectively, whether we are actively seeking it, or resisting with every bone in our body. Stagnant traditions or closely held beliefs that don't produce happy lives need to be examined and replaced with living tools that work.

In order to grow, we must be willing to give up the struggle to remain the same. You've heard the phrase "not being comfortable in your own skin." This growth process is about weaving the old with the new in order to experience renewal. By casting off the old skin, metaphorically speaking, we release our old ways of thinking and emerge with fresh new skin allowing doors to open for new beginnings.

Easy? No. Essential to happiness? Yes!

So as we stand on the leading edge of creation, in our individual lives and as a planet of consciousness, holding onto anything that prevents us from transforming makes no sense. We have the opportunity to look at yoga as it applies to our lives today and utilize its tremendous tools and empowerment for a richer and deeper experience. The liberties I'm taking are geared for results. In order to make this work for you, take and apply what calls out to you and leave the rest for later or share with a friend.

Blind faith is not a prerequisite. The ensuing assertions can be tested in the laboratory of your own life. In fact, I encourage you to do just that!

Since you were drawn to this book, there is something special here for you - without a doubt. If you are new to yoga, read with an open mind and ask yourself - how do I make yoga work for me?

Allow me be your personal yoga guide. If you don't know how or where to start, together we can develop and implement a plan to support your journey. Maybe you've tried doing yoga in the past and didn't find the right teacher or didn't get the support that you needed.

Let's take it slow by starting with the principles. Alternatively, you can go directly to the chapter(s) that interest you most. I am here to inspire you and to offer specific direction to get you started down the path of yoga. I will share exactly how you can use a variety of practices - traditional and nontraditional - to lead you to sustainable health, happiness and an engaging, satisfying life. If you still have questions, use the links at the end of each chapter to take you deeper.

If you are a practicing yogi already, ask yourself if your current practice is working for you, and open yourself to any new paths that might be calling your name.

It is possible for you to find clarity, purpose and a comfortable rhythm to your life. There is a reliable system you can use to feel good, to ignite your inner inspiration and strengthen your ability to create the life you want.

The system is yoga.

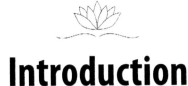

Introduction

*"I was BROKEN, overweight, out-of-shape,
defeated emotionally, spiritually and physically; stressed out
and I was ready to reinvent my life."*

- Laurie

Here is the way back to your authentic self, that part of you that is alive, healthy, powerful and filled with courage and passion. Remember that person?

It can be a deep plunge back to self. Somewhere in the process of living our lives, as we put our head down and charge forward, we end up in a place that surprises us. Often, it's not a good surprise.

We say to ourselves, "Wait a minute! This isn't what I thought my life would look like." It is almost like we have forgotten the truth of who we really are. We hunger for a life filled with meaning, health, freedom and happiness, but find ourselves living in ways that don't meet our deepest desires and with bodies filled with pain.

We want to feel healthy and vibrant, but our body isn't cooperating. Backs hurt, knees collapse, and joints ache. We feel tired and lack energy. My dad used to say, "The parts are wearing out!" Whether it is our body, mind or heart, we begin to feel disempowered and compromised. This place doesn't look like our dreams! Like Dorothy's adventure in Oz, it's a bit scary here because we don't know how to get back to feeling good.

Where do we turn for the healing and inspiration we need? Where are those ruby slippers??

The Yellow Brick Road

There is a path back. It is simple, but takes focus. For those who won't settle for a life that is uninspiring or a body that feels broken, the path of yoga is an answer that works. If you are a seeker, an adventurer in life, you want to be happier, healthier, and live authentically, then take this yogic map to guide you on your journey.

There was a time in my life where I felt as lost as Dorothy. I lacked direction and every path I explored was missing an essential ingredient for my health and happiness. My hands and feet were beginning to ache with the beginnings of arthritis. I loved being healthy and active, and I was determined to find a way to remain that way.

I have always been interested in health and fitness, as well as personal development and living a conscious, happy life, so when I was first introduced to yoga, it was a natural fit. However, I never would have believed just how much yoga would change my life!

Through yoga, my arthritis pain has vanished, and my body is stronger and healthier than it was when I was 20 years old. I've been able to magnetize rewarding lifework and meaningful connection to others. I've developed a deep understanding of what is truly important to me and become able to exercise my ability to powerfully direct my life into areas of greater joy.

The simple practices which we will explore in the following chapters will help you heal, too. I'll show you how to examine your habits and choose a path to healing. It is usually our fears and unhealthy patterns that contribute to the pain in our bodies and our lives. It is time to start down the road to healing.

It's time for something to change. Perhaps everything will change.

PART ONE

MIND BODY SOUL SPIRIT

Forget about enlightenment. Sit down wherever you are and listen to the wind that is singing in your veins. Feel the love, the longing, and the fear in your bones. Open your heart to who you are, right now, not who you would like to be. Not the saint you're striving to become. But the being right here before you, inside you, around you. All of you is holy. You're already more and less than whatever you can know. Breathe out, look in, let go.

- John Welwood

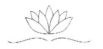

Chapter One

The Yoga Solution

*"What lies behind us and what lies before us
are tiny matters compared to what lies within us."*

- Ralph Waldo Emerson

My Story

I was introduced to yoga in a drafty gym in the depths of a harsh Chicago winter. My body shivered, but my spirit glowed! It was the perfect fit - a complement to my lifetime study of health, fitness, and personal growth.

Shortly after that first yoga class, I made the decision that this is what I wanted to do. I wanted to teach yoga.

I had never heard of the law of attraction, which is the universal principle that a vibration, whether it is a brain wave or electromagnetic heart vibration, will attract, like a magnet does, similar vibrations and opportunities. I just knew that I was very sure I wanted to do this yoga thing, and I knew I was on the right track.

The law of attraction kicked in and opportunity opened up for me when my teacher, Robin, asked me if I wanted to join her small staff and take over teaching her Thursday class. It was a tiny class of three dedicated students which she didn't have the heart to cancel. For me, it was quite an honor and a challenge to lead these three dedicated yogis: Dana, Amy and Liz. We practiced in a local synagogue by the altar. Perfect.

Somehow they stayed with me, and our yoga group, called Yoga Here and Now, grew. As I taught, I learned about the ways yoga heals and inspires.

We wanted to find a larger studio space, and once again, our desires opened a door when a local wellness center invited the original group of three teachers and their staff of one (me) to create a yoga program in their beautiful new million dollar addition. Law of attraction works again!

So, Yoga Here and Now went over there and became Avani Yoga with a large following of dedicated yogis.

In those days, you could be a yoga teacher just because you said you were. As yoga grew and was incorporated into gyms and wellness centers, there was a definite need for certification of some kind. Things were changing and studios everywhere began to require that their teachers had the basic certification, which is 200 hours of specialized training.

It was interesting to see the reactions I received when I told people I was going to become a certified yoga teacher. My students looked at me and asked, "Why?" To them it didn't matter if I had the papers or not - I was their teacher.

One acquaintance, a former yoga teacher herself, tried to dissuade me saying that there were already more yoga teachers than there were classes to fill them and that the field was already saturated. I knew right then that my future depended on what I chose to focus on and believe. I had a choice to drop into negativity and doubt or remain true to the conviction of my heart. My positive mindset and emotions ignited a vibration that had to be fulfilled. From then, I've never looked back and every yoga door I've ever knocked on, figuratively and literally, has opened to welcome me in.

To fulfill my training requirements, I decided the best option was an intensive yoga certification - a six week program, Monday through Friday. Because of the time requirement, I knew I would be taking time off from my other job and decided that if I was taking six weeks off to study, I would do it in an interesting place.

Since India was not an option for me at the time, I traveled to New York City to become certified in a Jivamukti style program. This style of yoga drew me because it's an active, athletic style with a focus on spiritual teachings and music. And New York drew me because, well, it's New York!

After returning home to Chicago, I resumed teaching in the hospital-affiliated health center with the same wonderful group of teachers. It was a certified Kripalu studio, but with a mixed style of teachers and class types. We all welcomed the diversity and learned from each other. Mostly, I learned from them.

Over the years, I've studied with yogis from many different styles and schools of thought. I guess I've morphed into a new age yogi, weaving together old and new, shedding skins that don't fit anymore to become comfortable in the skin I'm continually growing into.

As I've deepened my own practice of yoga, I've deepened in my understanding and belief in the Law of Attraction and how it is intertwined with the philosophy of the ancient yoga texts. Not every yogi will agree with me on that.

But everywhere the message is the same - yoga heals.

Yoga is a powerful tool to heal our body and transform our life. It's a doorway, an entry point that leads us toward awareness, freedom and peace. How does it do this?

Through the practice.

As a yoga instructor, I have worked with hundreds of people and witnessed their transformation as they applied certain principles in their lives. It usually begins with the desire to relieve pain or stress and create a healthier body and lifestyle. And then the magic begins.

It feels like magic because through this practice, unseen and unseemly parts of ourselves appear and then become transformed into something new. Voila! Aches, pains, and the effects of stress begin to diminish.

Not Just Posing

Put aside your preconceptions about yoga. This certainly isn't about touching your toes or standing on your head. We are going to explore an ancient tradition in a new, dynamic way. This is a way that will work for you, wherever you are in life, whatever your beliefs.

It is helpful to think of yoga as a metaphor.

Working with the outer body is also an opportunity to work with the inner self. We are not just stretching hamstrings - we are tuning in to ourselves to detect the tightness in our hearts or minds. Focusing attention on our body trains us to focus attention on our inner life experience. Looking for space in our hips, or spaces in between our breaths, teaches us to look for breathing space in our closest most volatile relationships. Investigating our discomfort in a challenging pose translates to investigating our discomfort in speaking our truth. Everything in yoga is geared toward change and growth, whether you are nineteen or ninety.

So, if you think that yoga is just stretching or navel gazing and chanting, then let me introduce you to my yoga. Vibrant, challenging, healing. Ancient yoga is for today and is just as cutting edge relevant in our modern world as it was when it was conceived. It will give you valuable tools to manage stress and will be a powerful, all encompassing practice that can touch every area of your life.

Visit **www.CatherineMazurYoga.com/solution**
to begin your yoga journey.

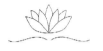

Chapter Two
What Is Yoga?

"And the day came when the risk to remain tight inside the bud was more painful than the risk it took to blossom."

\- Anais Nin

Harv's Story

Harv is there on his mat at the back of the class every week, rain or shine. He is about six foot four and as tight as a drum. But that's just his body- his mind is open and loose, and he's about the friendliest guy you'd ever want to know. At the end of practice, he's the first to say, "Thanks! Great class!" with an enthusiasm that inspires all of us. He inspires me. I think he inspires everyone whose life he touches.

From what I hear, he talks up yoga in the locker room after class every week, encouraging the guys to give yoga a try.

"Yoga is the best thing you can possibly do for your body. Don't worry if you're not flexible or if your hamstrings are tight. Yoga isn't for the flexible - it's for the inflexible - This is exactly what you need!" Harv relays his commentary to me afterwards.

Harv wasn't always a yoga fanatic. In fact, for many years he would never try anything unless he would excel. He was a super achiever, class valedictorian, and star athlete. He had a very narrow focus because he would only attempt things he knew he could master. Driven by some internal force, he could accept nothing but perfection from himself. He had a successful law practice, but was so inflexible with himself that he missed out on many opportunities and experiences by living a very rigid, self-restricted life.

When Harv's marriage failed, it put him into a tailspin. He entered therapy to help him sort things out. In the process, he came face to face with his fears and how they controlled his actions. He realized just how much he had lived by outer influences, so much that he never checked in with his deepest desires to see what he wanted from life. He was so preoccupied with appearances and perfection that he missed out on the juiciness in life that comes from trying something outside his comfort level. In time, his narrow focus on perfection began to soften and his options for life began to widen. He relaxed his unrealistic standards for himself and began to try things that really challenged him - including yoga.

Pushing himself into areas where he was uncomfortable opened up a whole new world; with it came a deep love of life. With his new found flexibility and acceptance of himself, he lives vibrantly and fully. Now Harv's mantra is, "Anything worth doing is worth doing poorly." In his 70s, he does the things he loves, whether he shines at them or shakes.

Not Just For The Young And Flexible

The number one thing that I hear when I tell people I teach yoga is, "I'm not flexible; I can't even touch my toes!"

Many people are surprised to learn that yoga is not about being flexible enough to touch your toes. Instead, it's about being flexible enough to look at yourself in a new way, stretching the whole of you so that every part of you feels good, healthy, happy and whole...not just your hamstrings.

Yoga is not just an exercise program. It is a method for healing your body, and can also be an entire philosophy for life.

It is a guidebook to point us in the direction of a meaningful life, happy, strong and calm.

Yoga is a healing system of theory and practice, a comprehensive system for finding health and happiness. The purpose of yoga is to create strength, awareness and harmony in both the mind and body. It is a physical, mental, and energetic discipline that aims to transform body and mind. There is a reason why yoga has been around for thousands of years. Its life changing ability is subtle, yet so powerful.

It's Not Religion

Thousands of years ago, a group of people decided to figure out a way to be the healthiest and happiest humans that they could be. Like our healthcare system today, their system wasn't working for them either. So, they set out to experiment and over time developed the ancient seeds of what has grown into the yoga that we know today.

This simple search for peace and health became widespread and continued to morph and grow through the decades and centuries. Through the years, yoga has been adopted by many diverse cultures and endorsed by different religions; however, this comprehensive system stands apart from any religious affiliation.

Its roots are deep and it has many, many branches. It is not a religion, but rather a way to balance our human experience through principles and practices that can be used by anyone, no matter their culture and beliefs.

The essence of yoga remains the same despite outward associations with any culture or tradition. It is possible to peel away all that has been overlaid, whether Sanskrit terms or Hindu philosophy, from the fundamentals of the practice and still use yoga's basic principles without needing to follow any of the various brandings over the years.

Whether or not yoga is a religion continues to be a highly debated topic, to me, the focus needs to be on the fact that yoga leads to healing, self knowledge and peace. Isn't this the original objective of most organized religions?

Beneath the differences in traditions and schools of thought, yoga is union. The word "yoga" actually means union. Coming from the root word, yuj, which means to yoke or join, yoga is above all else a union of body, mind and spirit.

A Vehicle For Transformation

Yoga is like an automobile. It takes us where we want to go. Our auto can be a Honda, Buick, or Saab. They all use similar technology to get us from our house to the grocery store, just as religion is a vehicle for spiritual enlightenment, whether it's Christianity, Buddhism or Islam.

It is a vehicle to steer us into health and a fulfilled life no matter what our belief system. The applied principles, or the "technology" of yoga, will steer us toward happiness, health and personal growth, just as surely as a map and a car can bring us to the destination of our choice. So, jump on in and let's get going on the road to a fulfilled, pain free, happy, healthy life!

To get help getting your yoga car started and to learn yoga basics, visit **www.CatherineMazurYoga.com/starthere**

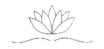

Chapter Three

51 Yoga Benefits

"Yoga is not about touching your toes.
It's about what you learn on the way down."

- Unknown

Laurie's Story

It was back in December 2010, and Laurie had just left a high stress traveling job. She was in her second year of rehab after a major life-changing foot surgery which led to a stroke. She was overweight, out of shape, and defeated emotionally, spiritually and physically.

Laurie was ready to reinvent her life when she went to her first yoga class with me. She told me years later that she knew she was in for something hard - but good. Over the course of 12 months, she was a regular in class. She began to be inspired. She redirected her life in a much more positive direction. She swam, ran and worked out. Over time, things totally turned around for her. Of all those activities, her yoga classes provided her with most life changing lessons that ultimately changed the direction of her life.

Yoga can change your life, too. It can inspire you and empower you to grow and stretch in ways that you never imagined; powerful ways that turn out to be the very things that you need. Like Laurie's estimation of her yoga classes, hard - but good.

Below are 51 of the benefits that are often associated with a regular yoga practice.

Physical Benefits

1. Back pain relief

    I am placing back pain relief at the top of the list because it is the number one benefit my students report.

    Most minor back pain comes from inactivity and lifestyle. Unfortunately, we spend most of our time sitting. We sit and sip our morning coffee, we sit in the car on the way to work, class or appointments, and sit again once we arrive.

    During the day, we might get up and walk around for a brief time, but then we sit again, even through lunch breaks. The great majority of us spend our days sitting at the computer, sitting behind the wheel, and then sitting on the sofa to relax, exhausted by all that sitting.

    Our bodies were not meant for all of this sitting! It is the single major cause of back pain and conditions which cause compression in the spine.

    Over time, yoga will increase your strength and flexibility, and effectively counteract the tightness and the weak muscles that are the result of our seated lifestyle.

2. Better alignment of the spine

    When the spine is correctly aligned, it relieves back pain. The standing poses, as well as many of the seated poses, help to develop core strength which holds the spine in better alignment.

3. Increases muscle strength and tone

   Standing poses, balance poses, and an active style of yoga, such as vinyasa, require muscular engagement and endurance. The beauty of yoga is that it develops muscle strength in a balanced fashion, strengthening the large opposing muscle groups and toning the supporting ones.

4. Cardio health

   As we engage the large muscles of the body, our heart rate rises to meet the increased demand for oxygen to be sent to the muscles. This strengthens the heart muscle and improves cardiac health.

5. Circulatory health

   Doing the poses increases heart rate and, as our heart rate is elevated, the lungs work harder to supply more oxygen. Breath deepens and lung capacity increases, contributing to the overall health of our circulatory system.

6. Increases blood flow

   Increased heart rate will increase our blood flow. This is beneficial for our organs and circulatory system.

7. Increases flexibility

   All the stretching done in the poses increases flexibility. The by product of flexibility is a limber body, less at risk of injury from pulled or strained muscles. Flexible muscles will allow us a larger range of motion, affecting our ability to perform daily functions and adding to our quality of life.

8. Joint health

    As the muscles become balanced and strong, our joints are more fully protected. The movements stimulate the lymphatic system which ultimately reduces inflammation in the body and swelling in the joints.

9. Improves arthritis

    It is possible to get relief from some forms of arthritis through the regular practice of yoga. With our internal systems working together more effectively the nutrients are absorbed and waste products are eliminated more efficiently. This can result in reduced inflammation and pain relief.

10. Strengthens bones

    All weight bearing exercises improve bone density. With the variety of poses done on the forearms, hands, knees and feet, yoga is an excellent way to strengthen our entire skeletal system.

11. Improves respiration

    The yoga practice of breathing, called pranayama, is effective in clearing and relieving sinus pressure, along with the associated symptoms of nasal allergies. It increases lung capacity and function.

12. Improves overall spinal health

    With increased blood flow to the spine, spinal health increases. Yoga has been shown to help to correct spinal conditions like scoliosis, lordosis and kyphosis. With modifications and a gentle, prudent approach, even a beginner yogi can benefit. These conditions, as well as stenosis and problems with the intervertebral disks, can be improved.

13. Improves lymph flow

    In yoga, all muscles, both commonly used major and seldom used minor muscles, are utilized. This contributes to increased lymph fluid flow. Lymph fluid, unlike blood, does not have a pump to move it throughout the body. The lymph system, whose function is to carry away waste products from the cells, is an extensive system of tiny channels running throughout the body. The lymph system depends on muscular action to move this lymph fluid along the channels. As we practice yoga, the muscles' squeezing action acts to initiate flow of fluid through the lymph ducts and channels.

Additionally the inversions, such as headstands or legs up the wall, help to drain lymph fluid from the lower extremities.

14. Lowers blood pressure

Inversions can effectively lower blood pressure. Small sensors called baroreceptors are located in the base of our throat. These baroreceptors measure the blood pressure in the body regulating it. When the legs are elevated above the heart it causes a flood of blood draining towards these receptors. When this rise in the blood pressure is detected by these sensors they respond with a signal to the body. Upon detecting this heightened blood pressure, the baroreceptors moderate the flow to reduce blood pressure.

15. Balances blood sugar

New research shows that just 15 minutes of exercise a day can increase lifespan by years. Now a small study published in the journal *Diabetes Care* has uncovered the benefits of gentle yoga on type two diabetes. In a study involving diabetics with one group doing yoga three times a week and the control group doing no added activity, the blood glucose levels of the people in the yoga group held steady, while the levels of those in the control group rose.

16. Weight reduction

Some forms of yoga provide a level of exercise which increases the calorie burn. The ratio of physical activity which expends calories to our calorie intake each day determines whether we maintain, gain or lose weight. Muscles, even in their resting state, will burn more calories than fat. So, as we develop more muscle fiber and lose fat, our metabolism will burn more calories even in inactivity.

17. Protection from injury

The increased flexibility, balance, and joint stabilization which comes from our yoga practice helps protect us from falls and strains.

18. Improves athletic performance

With less injury, increased balance and flexibility athletic performance is enhanced.

19. Balances adrenals and hormones

Yoga is a great stress reliever. When anxiety and a constant state of stress exist for a prolonged period, it is common to experience adrenal fatigue. Disrupted sleep, lack of energy, and other symptoms are often the result of overworked adrenal glands. When the adrenals are overworked they can lose their ability to do their job which can also lead to mood swings, lack of energy, and infertility.

20. Improves posture

With increased body awareness and stronger back muscles, posture improves. The very nature of yoga teaches one to hold their body in a healthier alignment.

21. Balances metabolism

Yoga can be a great way to increase metabolism. It improves digestion and circulation and increases lean muscle mass which will burn more calories. Any physical activity and sustained movement can increase metabolic rate.

22. Improves immune function

Yoga practice has frequently been correlated with a stronger immune system. This is in part because of its ability to reduce the effects of tension and stress. Also, it improves lymph function which is essential to the immune system's effectiveness.

23. Improves energy levels

Everything about yoga will improve your energy. The practice of physical yoga is intended to open the meridians of energy in the body and energize your metabolism. The breathing exercises will oxygenate your cells. Dealing with stress, worry, depression and anger takes up great amounts of energy. As you learn new mental habits, this energy is freed up to be used in other areas of your life.

24. Improves nervous system function

In our society, most of us deal with constant stress. When this occurs, our nervous system gets stuck in the fight or flight syndrome. The two branches of the nervous system, sympathetic and parasympathetic, are designed to balance each other out. The sympathetic side is activated when a potentially dangerous situation arises. The endocrine system will pump hormones into the bloodstream to ramp up the heart rate to oxygenate the muscle for action. Blood pressure rises and breathing gets stronger.

This is great if we need to run from a tiger...but not if it is a sustained state produced by everyday stress. Our ancestors' nervous systems automatically returned to a normal resting state when the immediate danger passed. They didn't stay in fight or flight syndrome because their parasympathetic nervous system brought them back into balance. In a healthy state, when the stressor is gone, the brain releases neurotransmitters to the body to lower our heart rate and relax our muscles.

Due to the level of stress in today's world, the two sides of our nervous system are not balanced. Once the adrenals become exhausted from continually dumping cortisol into the system, the immune system is compromised which leads to a compromised functioning of the nervous system. The practice of yoga and its ability to reduce the effects of stress will help to balance these two important branches of our central nervous system

25. Increases lung capacity

The yoga practices of working with breath greatly increase breath control, depth and effective oxygenation. An added benefit is increased lung capacity.

26. Promotes healthier connective tissue

As joints get support from the surrounding muscles, it protects the ligaments and tendons from being strained.

27. Improves balance

If we don't use it, we lose it - this goes for balance, as well as everything else. Many yoga poses focus on balancing, which continues to increase as we practice. Balance poses strengthen the small stabilizer muscles of the joints, ankles, knees, hips and spine.

28. Reduces belly fat

There has been shown to be a correlation between levels of stress, heightened cortisol levels and abdominal fat. As we learn to manage stress through the practice of yoga, we reverse this trend.

29. Improves digestion

Because the majority of the digestive tract is located in the abdomen, yoga poses that focus on the core will help the organs function properly. Twisting poses help wring out the digestive tract and detoxify the organs.

30. Gastrointestinal function improves

The poses have been shown to improve GI function in both men and women who practice yoga. Compressing and twisting the organs of elimination relieves problems with diarrhea, gas and intestinal pain.

31. Improves sex

Yoga helps to improve one's sensitivity and relieves tension and stress. These alone can improve your sex life. More importantly, yoga strengthens the pelvic floor muscles, increases energy, endurance and flexibility.

32. Enhances sleep

A well documented fact is that yoga calms the nervous system. The stress hormone, cortisol, comes into balance and the endocrine system works properly. With hormones balanced and stress relieved, we are able to relax and get a good night sleep.

Mental Benefits

33. Promotes mental clarity

When the effects of stress are alleviated, we are able to think more clearly. Also, heightened levels of oxygen from yogic breathing feed the brain. Lung capacity increases and the benefit of more oxygen is greater mental clarity.

34. Improves memory

Improved blood circulation to the brain, as well as the reduction in stress, will result in a better memory. Learning to focus your mind in meditation improves memory function.

35. Attention span improves

Focused breathing and meditation will sharpen your ability to stay focused in other areas of life. Also, training the brain to listen closely for the verbal cues given during a yoga class will lengthen your attention span.

36. Heightens awareness

A natural byproduct of the inner and outer work of yoga is mental clarity. The combination of poses and other mindfulness practices produce a level of awareness of body and mind. We begin to see things with a more realistic perspective.

37. Heightens self-esteem

As we see things more holistically and realistically, it leads to a higher self esteem. Mastering the poses and improving our strength and balance improves the way we feel about ourselves. The purpose of yoga is to clear away the misconceptions we have about our true nature. We begin to see the perfection of everything, including ourselves.

38. Heightens inner strength

Focusing the mind in meditation requires concentration. With sustained practice, it will increase our willpower, leading to inner strength.

39. Increases focus

The practices of sensory withdrawal, concentration and meditation develop our mental faculties and ability to maintain focus for extended periods of time. This ability spills over into every area of our life.

Emotional Benefits

40. Increases happiness and contentment

All of the above results in feeling more well-adjusted, happy and free. Through meditation and the study of yogic principles, we learn to recognize what is important in life and our perspective shifts on many levels, bringing us peace, contentment and bliss.

41. Promotes calm

With our hormones in balance, our blood pressure reduced, increased awareness and a larger perspective on our lives, we more readily remain calm in the face of life's challenges.

42. Balances mood and emotional swings

With our new tools for stress relief and management, our emotional state is greatly improved. The mental practices enable us to level out the highs and lows as we experience equanimity.

43. Relieves anxiety

The practice of controlled breathing, or pranayama, used in yoga will reduce anxiety. The physical practice helps to dispel the worry and stress that are the underlying causes of anxiety.

44. Relieves depression

Emotional and/or mental upheaval, whether it's stress, depression, or anxiety are often the result of long-term tension patterns. These patterns can create blockages in our energy flow. Yoga helps us discover greater emotional well-being by releasing tension and dissolving the emotional blocks that hold us back from living a happy, healthy life. Breath and targeted movement provide physical benefits as well as mood benefits. Specific poses, such as backbending, have been documented to provide physical benefits and mood benefits to individuals suffering from chronic depression.

Spiritual Benefits

45. Grounding

The poses, particularly savasana, contribute to a heightened sense of security and foundation. The entire practice is meant to return the practitioner to their deepest roots.

46. Self acceptance

Through yoga practice, one learns that perfection is not the goal of the poses, but instead the focus is to develop self awareness, appreciation and self acceptance.

47. Positive energy levels improve

When we are not constantly bombarded by the effects of stress and physical ailments, it frees up tremendous storehouses of energy that were previously used to deal with our struggles, suffering and pain. When we begin to focus our energies toward growth and positive thoughts, we retrain ourselves to maintain a positive outlook.

48. Renewed purpose and personal responsibility

With a dedicated yoga practice, we regain our vitality and a renewed sense of purpose. We see ourselves as part of the larger community of mankind and step up into responsible action.

49. Social skills improve

In yoga, we learn the interconnectedness of all of life. Our yoga practice evolves from a personal journey to one that connects us to the community. We become better parents, partners, and community members.

50. Personal guidance system improves

Immersed in the practice and principles of yoga and surrounded by the enlightened community of yogis, we are able to tap into our inner guidance system and live a meaning filled life.

51. Heightens passion for life

The practice of turning inward and focusing on the deeper meaning of life through meditation and self study will ignite our passion to live a life of meaning.

By now you're getting the idea that yoga is good for you. Not just for your body, but for mind, soul, and spirit. Maybe you know this already from personal experience and have discovered that it makes you feel better on many levels. I'd love to hear your story. Share it with me by visiting my website.

By focusing on breath, poses and meditation, our regular yoga practice creates mental clarity and calmness, increases body awareness, heals the body, relieves chronic stress patterns, relaxes the mind, centers attention, and sharpens concentration.

Learn how 18 people broke through to obtain life changing benefits at **www.CatherineMazurYoga.com/stories**

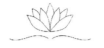

Chapter Four

Healing Hearts And Backs

"To live in this world you must be able to do three things:
to love what is mortal;
to hold it against your bones knowing
your own life depends on it; and,
when the time comes to let it go, to let it go."
- Mary Oliver

Val's Story

Val had been through a rough few years. When her very healthy dad suddenly became ill and rapidly declined, she made the decision to leave her home in California and move across the country to Pennsylvania to be his primary caregiver. She had always been extremely close to her parents and wanted to do everything she could to help.

A year later, he passed away after a courageous battle with cancer, Val by his side every day. Four months later, she lost her mom to pneumonia. Being the primary caretaker for her parents and then losing both of them within the same year, left her feeling like an orphan. *She had yet to realize the extent of the toll it took on her.*

Later that year, her company experienced a major reorganization and she was laid off, only eight short months after losing her father and four months after losing her mom. What could happen next?

Completely broken and unable to process her profound grief, she struggled with so much loss in such a short period of time. As each day passed, the grief she couldn't process started manifesting in her body. She was experiencing excruciating back pain, sciatica, lethargy, and insomnia, and her depression was like a black hole.

A former athlete, Val was reduced to wearing a back brace for support and most days stayed in bed and cried; spirit broken and mind unraveling.

Trying to heal her back pain, she regularly visited her chiropractor to get some relief. However, the adjustments never held for very long and she would again find herself paralyzed with pain when her back or neck went out of alignment. Her chiropractor suggested that there seemed to be something else going on in her body and energy field.

Low back pain is often related to emotional issues, and Val felt in her heart that he was right. With all that she had emotionally gone through in the previous years, she wondered if it might be an energy blockage that needed to be addressed by another modality.

In a perfect sequence of events, orchestrated by a benevolent universe, Val and I met and began an amazing journey together, focusing on healing yoga sessions for her back, along with energy healing for her soul.

Over the course of a year, she slowly mended her body and heart. The yoga sessions relieved her back spasms and her body became strong again. At the same time, we focused on the internal practices of yoga, using meditation, energy work and self inquiry to shift the energy that was keeping her stuck in depression and pain.

Her experience of healing was so profound that she decided to deepen her knowledge of yoga and committed to an extensive 200 hour training to become a certified yoga instructor.

Now, Val uses her knowledge and personal experience to teach the healing power of yoga to others.

Val's story illustrates how everything is interrelated - physical pain, emotional pain and mental pain are bound together in mysterious ways. Our every thought and action creates a reaction. We need to learn the right attitude and actions to take care of our bodies, hearts and brains. When we find the balance that keeps us happy and healthy, our energy flows freely. Stuck energy, as Val learned, can be the source of much suffering.

In the following chapters, you will learn:

- How to release stuck energy in your body
- Physical yoga poses to heal your body and your heart
- How to be proactive for your health
- How to take right action in the world

Four paths can be taken. Any one of them, and all of them, can be the healing answer that you are looking for. They are the path of knowledge, the path of action, the path of devotion and the royal path of meditation.

For a mind expanding game that Val used to help her find her path, visit **www.CatherineMazurYoga.com/val**

Chapter Five

Four Paths For Healing

*"You have a wellspring of beautiful energy inside of you.
When you are open you feel it;
when you are closed you don't."*

- Michael Singer, *The Untethered Soul*

It's Elemental

Think back to chemistry class when you learned about the basic building blocks in our DNA. Been a long time since high school? That's okay, me too.

We are made from four essential elements, inseparable in our human existence.

These four elements are carbon, hydrogen, oxygen and nitrogen. Each of these elements shows up in our world as earth, fire, water and air.

- Carbon relates to earth
- Hydrogen relates to fire
- Oxygen relates to water
- Nitrogen relates to air

As humans, we are also composed of four basic components which are mind, body, soul, and spirit.

In the system of yoga, there are four main paths. Jnana yoga, the path of knowledge; Karma yoga, the path of action, Bhakti yoga, the path of devotion; Raja yoga, path of meditation.

Although these four paths are interrelated, their focus is different. We are different in the way we approach and experience the world, we have our own preferred style of learning. We are interested in different paths and life experiences. How boring it would be if we all were the same! We need the combination of elements to create a dynamic whole.

Which Path Is Calling You?

There's a yoga path that is custom tailored for each of us. These four paths relate to the four different aspects of human life which are mind, body, soul or heart, and spirit and their corresponding elements of earth, fire, water and air.

The path of the knowledge, Jnana yoga is solid like the earth. It is what you think.

The path of action, Karma yoga is dynamic like fire. It is what you do.

The path of devotion, Bhakti yoga is flowing like water. It is what you are committed to.

The path of meditation, Raja yoga is ethereal like air. It is what you are.

Of course, each of us has elements of all types within us, just as we are made of all four of the essential building blocks for our DNA, but we generally lead with a certain type of energy and focus. Which path draws you most: Jnana, Karma, Bhakti, or Raja?

The Mind Path, Jnana Yoga, Earth

Some people are mentally orientated and very analytical. They love the path of knowledge and learning. They want facts and a logical explanation for everything. Looking for proof and a solid foundation beneath their beliefs and what they choose, they are earth element types.

Factual details and history appeal to them. They love a mental challenge and are prolific readers, scholars and lifelong learners. The programs and podcasts they listen to are geared to educate and inform them, and from this vantage point, they choose the direction of their life. Thinkers and lovers of knowledge will be naturally drawn to Jnana yoga, the path of knowledge.

The Action Path, Karma Yoga, Fire

Action oriented people are always moving and doing. Like the jumping flames of a fire, they are always reaching for the next experience. They are adventurers who push forward with fiery energy to get to work and get it done. Living with passion and substantial energy, they often have many balls in the air.

They move projects forward to get results and make a difference. Because they blaze a trail, these people are often viewed as leaders in their community or field of expertise. Naturally, those who value action and results will be drawn to the path of Karma yoga, the path of action.

The Heart Path, Bhakti Yoga, Water

Others lead with the heart and approach life in an emotional way. They are sensitive, with a great awareness for others. They wait for their heart to lead them, and then follow its urging. Rather than pushing for action or analyzing the facts, they prefer to flow with their intuition. They are gentle and relaxed in their orientation to learning and life.

People who follow this path of heart are devoted to their choices, ideals and values. They support their bodies and minds and follow through with their well informed choices about their health. Their inner world needs to be aligned with their outer world, so they often look for a certain internal sign before making a decision.

Feeling comfortable is important to them, not just in their body, but in their life plan, as they fluidly feel their way through to the next step in life. Once they determine what that path is, their devotion runs deep, like the ocean. These individuals will find the path of Bhakti yoga, devotion, draws their heart.

The Path Of Meditation, Raja Yoga, Air

There is one more element, air. Expansive thinking people who have upward energy and are open to new possibilities are hungry seekers. They live on a large scale, reflecting on the bigger picture. Dreamers and philosophers, they are explorers of the unseen and unknown. Thought leaders, inventors and Nobel Prize winners; they are people who don't look at what is impossible, but for what might be possible. The entire universe is their playing field and great ideas are born out of their unlimited type of thinking. They are disciplined with their physical body as well as their mind, knowing that the two are intimately connected. Raja yoga, the path of meditation, appeals to their sense of inquisitiveness and possibility. They see it as a path to explore the inner recesses of the mind and the outer limits of the universe.

These four paths are intertwined through the traditions and types of yoga. Many yogis don't even realize there are four main paths, they just know that some aspects of yoga draw them more than others. Although each of us will benefit from all of these paths of yoga, we will find ourselves drawn more toward one of these particular paths, depending on our nature and what we enjoy in life.

Discover your path at
www.CatherineMazurYoga.com/mypath

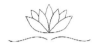

Chapter Six

Four Principles For Happiness

*"The real mission you have in life is
to make yourself happy,
and in order to be happy,
you have to look at what you believe."*

- Miguel Ruiz,
*The Mastery of Love:
A Practical Guide to the Art of Relationship*

I love the book *The Four Agreements*, by Miguel Ruiz. It's a classic. In it, he tells us of four powerful agreements that we can make with our self that can change our life.

I understand them as the following:

- **Question your conclusions**. It might astonish you to realize how much of your thinking is an assumption. We assume things all day long, such as that our car will always start or our favorite Starbucks will be open. When we are wrong - it doesn't and it isn't - it upsets us. Rightly so. These assumptions help us to lead a sane and predictable life. Although these beliefs are benign, if we look deeper we can see them as part of a habitual way of thinking which we all practice. This way of thinking causes us pain. The small assumptions are merely annoying. It's the larger underlying assumptions we have about life that causes our bigger suffering. We assume someone is mad at us, or that we have let someone down. We assume we should be happier and life should be easier. We suffer needlessly from these assumptions. Assuming our children should act a certain way or believing that our spouse should be understanding at all times in order for us to be happy are assumptions that hurt. We suffer when we believe them. Question the beliefs that are at the root of your pain. Take a big step back and you begin to see you have a choice about the meaning you place on the events and circumstances of your life.

- **Choose your words carefully.** Before you speak, ask yourself, "Is it true? Is it kind? Is it necessary?" If you let this principle govern everything that comes out of your mouth, you will be a much happier person. You will be a more loyal friend and a better influence on everyone in your life. Once you begin to guard what you say, you will find it changes your life because when you begin to examine your words it leads you to examine your thoughts and beliefs. Try it and see for yourself. When you realize that your words are a reflection of your thoughts and that your thoughts create your future, you will start to pay attention to what comes through your lips.

If you know something hurtful
and not true, don't say it.
If you know something hurtful
and true, don't say it.
If you know something helpful
but not true, don't say it.
If you know something helpful
and true, find the right time to say it.

- The Buddha

- **Lighten up!** A great amount of suffering comes from thinking that other people's actions, reactions and comments are directed at you. It might really seem that way, but at the heart of the matter it's rarely about you, it's about them. We have the power to be in control of our reactions to anything and everything that occurs. We are all self absorbed to a certain extent, and the more we can let it go and not take everything so personally, the happier we will be. The truth is, we are all so wrapped up in our own "stuff" that we limit our possibilities. Our reactions are automatic and defensive to protect our egos. When we take a step back, stop assuming and don't take things as a personal affront, we get freedom to really notice the choices we have. We see how our defensive reactions impact the people around us and the direction of our life.

- **Be real.** When you know that you have done your best job possible and not let anything fall to the side, you feel great. The tricky part is honestly recognizing your capacity and determining the extent of your individual responsibility in any given situation. Sometimes the best you can do, the best choice, is to do nothing. Your best will vary from day to day, moment to moment, and is dependant on your health, emotional state, energy level and the unique situation you are faced with. It's important to be discerning in every situation because doing too much can be detrimental to your health and also can hurt others. When you enable others by doing too much for them, it can stunt their growth, ultimately making life harder for them - and sometimes for you! Always doing your best involves being present and conscious enough to discern what the best plan of action is; it could be taking a nap or running a marathon, depending on the day.

These four principles are powerful directives for our lives and relate to one of the different types of yoga. As we explore the four main paths of yoga in the following sections, we will take a closer look at ways which we can apply these four principles to our life and discover the powerful changes that they bring.

For practical help to apply the four principles
of happiness to your life, visit
www.CatherineMazurYoga.com/fourprinciples

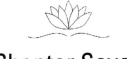

Chapter Seven

Basic Poses And Beyond

*"The most fortunate are those who have
a wonderful capacity to appreciate again and again,
freshly and naively, the basic goods of life,
with awe, pleasure, wonder and even ecstasy"*
- Abraham Maslow

*C*lass is underway and the students are moving through the yoga poses. This class is a sweaty, challenging vinyasa flow. The teacher leads us into a warrior pose and instructs us to hold it steady and breathe. And hold. And breathe. And hold. And breathe.

Leg muscles protest, but we are instructed to hold for another breath. As we hold the pose for an extra breath, we notice what we're feeling and then we notice how we react to that feeling. "It will pass," a small internal voice reassure us, "Stay, breathe, soften."

The teacher releases us to continue to flow. Whew! Made it. This, or some variation of it, is part of the process of yoga. Holding the poses and challenging our bodies also challenges our spirit. The greatest challenge is to remain aware to the raw sensations and moment *to moment breathing. Through this process we notice what we are feeling. More importantly, we begin to become aware of how we react to those thoughts and feelings. It is through this discipline that we learn to examine our beliefs and challenge ourselves to grow beyond our limiting beliefs and find our inner strength.*

At the studio down the street, the students are sitting on bolsters for the beginning of a restorative yoga class. The pace is slow and the focus is on meditation. The challenge here is to remain present and focused. As they are led through a guided meditation, minds begin to wander. "What will I make for dinner?", "I wonder why they never returned my call...", "I need new yoga pants." When the teacher encourages the release of thought, encouraging students to stay focused on the mantra, they are drawn back to their intended focus. Through this process, they gain awareness of the working of their mind - the crazy, wandering mind. The practice of meditation trains the mind, just as the physical practice trains the body. So simple, but so difficult!

A Few Basic Poses

There are over 50 types of yoga ranging from a sweaty power workout to a gentler, more meditative approach. All forms originated like branches from the same tree and continue to branch out further as new variations of yoga emerge.

Because there are so many different kinds of yoga practices, it is possible for anyone at any level to begin a yoga practice. The important thing is to find a practice that works for you.

It's beyond the scope of this book to delve into all the different styles, but below is a description of some of the most basic poses that you are likely to find in any yoga class.

In each of these poses, move slowly and breath deeply, releasing on your exhales. Hold each pose for 5-10 breaths. You can follow the video on my website, so that you can see the proper pose positions.

Child

One of the most basic poses is balasana, child pose. Come onto your hands and knees and begin to sit your hips back and down toward your heels. Stretch your arms forward and let your head and chest sink down toward the floor. If this bothers your neck, place a yoga block or a fist under your forehead for support. Continue to soften and relax, allowing your legs, hips, back, feet, and arms to release.

Cat Cow

Come back onto your hands and knees (this is commonly called tabletop). Your hands should be directly below your shoulders and your knees below your hips. Begin to exhale and round your back like a cat, tucking your tailbone under and your chin into your chest. Push your hands into the mat and keep your arms straight, with your belly drawing in and up towards your spine. Then, to move into cow pose, on your inhale slowly lift your chin and let your spine slump down toward the floor. Slide your shoulders away from your ears. Continue to move smoothly and slowly between these two poses, matching the movements to your inhales and exhales.

Spinal Extension

Begin on your hands and knees with your wrists directly under your shoulders and knees directly under your hips in tabletop. Keep your spine in its natural alignment, with your abdominal muscles engaged to support your low back. Gaze down, just in front of your fingertips so your head is aligned with the rest of your spine. Reach one arm forward, pinky finger toward the floor and thumb up, like a karate chop. Extend the opposite leg behind you, keeping it at hip height with your toes pointing down and flexing through the heel. Reach through your fingertips and heel of the foot simultaneously. Hold for 5 to 10 breaths and then switch sides.

Thread The Needle

Begin in tabletop. On an exhale, slide your right arm underneath your left arm with your palm facing up bringing your right shoulder all the way down towards the mat. If possible, rest your right ear and cheek on the mat looking towards your left. Do not press your weight into your head, instead adjust your position so you don't strain your neck or shoulder. Keep your hips raised. Soften and relax your lower back and allow all of the tension in your shoulders, arms and neck to drain away. Hold for 5 to 10 long, slow breaths and then gently release and switch sides.

Mountain

Standing at the front of your mat, press all four corners of your feet into the ground. Activate your legs by slightly lifting the arches of your feet and squeezing your thigh muscles to lift your kneecaps. Tone your low belly slightly and lift your ribcage out of your waistline. Roll your shoulders up, back and down, allowing your arms to hang loosely by your sides, pinky fingers rolling slightly in as thumbs slightly turn out. Your chin is parallel to the floor and draw back your ears to align the head directly atop the shoulders. If you want, sweep your arms up overhead while pressing your shoulders down and away from your ears.

Forward Fold

From mountain pose, hinge forward from the hips with your knees slightly bent. Let your arms hang long and loose and your head be heavy to release your neck muscles. Tone your belly to protect your low back. As the back of your body begins to release, you can gradually begin to straighten your legs.

Tree

Standing in mountain pose, shift your weight onto one foot and slide the other foot onto your ankle, calf or above the knee against your thigh. Pick a spot to look at and don't shift your eyes around. This gazing point is called a drishti and your steady gaze will help you stay balanced. You can use your arms to help you balance, bring your palms together at your heart, or raise your arms overhead.

Cobbler

From a seated position, bring the soles of your feet together and let your knees fall away from each other. Grasp your ankles or feet. Keep your low belly toned as you press your elbows down against the inner thighs. If you wish, lower your chin towards your chest and round your back, softening your shoulders away from your ears.

Bridge

Lower yourself onto your back and bend your knees, placing your feet flat on the floor. Your feet should be hip distance apart and either directly below your knees or slightly closer to your hips. With your arms by your sides, press into your feet to lift your hips off the floor. Relax the muscles in your rear end as you press into your heels to lift your spine up into your body. Lift your chin slightly away from your chest to keep the natural arch in the back of your neck. Do not flatten your neck against the floor. Feel the spine between your shoulder blades lifting your chest higher. After 5-10 breaths, slowly lower your back to the floor. Bridge pose can be repeated another time or two if you want. After your final bridge pose, wait for your back to release a bit and then hug your knees into your chest.

Supine Twist

Lying on your back, draw your knees up, around and into your ribs. Then open and extend your arms out to the side and onto the floor. Lower your bent knees toward your extended right arm, keeping them curled in and up as you slightly roll onto your side hip. The opposite arm remains open, reaching to the other side which will help to release your back ribs toward the floor. After 5-10 breaths, bring your legs back up, realign your spine and repeat the twist to the other side.

Savasana

Lying down on your back relax your entire body. Let your feet fall open and your legs and arms rest, palms facing up. If your lower back bothers you, slide a pillow, rolled blanket, or bolster underneath your knees. Close your eyes and let your head sink into the floor. Soften the muscles in your face, your eyes and your jaw. Release your shoulders, your low back, and let your breath be soft and easy. Stay here for 5-10 minutes, enjoying the rest.

Beyond The Poses

Beyond the poses lies the real power of yoga. When we notice our reactions as we are challenged to hold the poses, it creates an awareness. We come face to face with our edges. We notice our difficulty staying focused and to just stay, being present to whatever is arising in that very moment.

We were taught how to move and how to behave, but we were never taught how to be still and examine what's within. This is the true practice and power of yoga: finding the discipline we need to stay focused and learning to reach deep inside to find what is true for us. It begins with the movement, and then seeps into the stillness and slowly, we shift. Yoga requires that we get quiet and present enough to hear the voice of our heart. We begin to know ourselves in a way we've long forgotten. Or maybe never knew.

As we learn to listen to our bodies, it prepares the path for us to hear our thoughts and listen to our heart.

Want help with a basic pose sequencing flow?
Need inspiration to get on your mat? Visit
www.CatherineMazurYoga.com/poses

Chapter Eight
A New Story

"There are many forms of self we inhabit over a lifetime.
One self carries us to the extent of its usefulness and dies.
We are then forced to put that once beloved skin to rest,
to join it with the ground of spirit so it may fertilize
the next skin of self that will carry us into tomorrow.
There is always grief for what is lost and always surprise
at what is to be born. But much of our pain in living
comes from wearing a dead and useless skin,
refusing to put it to rest. We live, embrace, and put to rest
our dearest things, including how we see ourselves,
so we can resurrect our lives anew."

- Mark Nepo, *The Book of Awakening*

Sherry's Story

Sherry wanted to be a giver. She told me, "I struggle with believing
in myself, doubting that I have anything valuable to give. Over time,
I've begun to believe that life is a struggle and I should just settle and
not even expect to have it all. Then I ask myself - why did I adopt that
belief? How did I get from the unbridled optimism of my childhood
into the cynicism of my adulthood?"

When we were children, we were experts in happiness. (And really flexible, too!)

We knew what we wanted and what we were passionate about. Fun, laughter and self direction came naturally for us. Babies and toddlers delight in sensations, exploring their world, expressing their needs openly, smiling and laughing easily. Happiness is our natural state.

From Inner Focus To Outer Focus

Children are sponges, soaking up subtle hints and messages from the world around them. They interpret and form beliefs by looking at other people's reactions. In order to be accepted, as children we adopt our parents' values and opinions. This causes a chain effect as we look to the outer world to define ourselves, instead of looking inward and feeling our creative brilliance and inner joy.

We are taught that our report card defines our value and are conditioned to believe that our popularity determines our worth. These beliefs shape our inner reality which in turn creates our outer reality. Instead of living from the inside out, we shape our lives from the outside in.

The human experience is a kaleidoscope of external experiences and in turn, our internal reactions to them. These reactions form our beliefs. Our beliefs become the paradigm that we live by. Our paradigm steers the course of our life and drives our behavior which determines our results over our lifetime.

Deep in our subconscious mind, we form the belief that life is a struggle and we shouldn't expect to be happy and fulfilled. We believe the untruth that we can't live with purpose and authenticity and be financially successful. Our programmed subconscious mind holds the belief that life is hard, we can't have it all, or we shouldn't expect too much, we aren't really up to the task. Not good enough, smart enough, or talented enough. With this as our core belief, we create a reality that reflects that.

Wake Up!

We don't even recognize the limiting and self deprecating thoughts that we are thinking or fully realize the impact our own words have on us. So we tell ourselves things that aren't very kind. Mean things.

We are quick to think, *How could I say that - I am such an idiot!* or *I don't have what it takes - what's wrong with me?* We would never say these things to a friend, but here we are saying them to ourselves over and over. We are prey to self doubts and criticism about our accomplishments and abilities. Stuck in patterns that often have their roots in our childhood, we continue to seek approval from others at the expense of ourselves.

Whether we are consciously berating ourselves for saying something stupid or subconsciously comparing our sales reports or earning ability to others, we must monitor our thoughts because thoughts are the words we feed our mind.

Listen carefully. Be aware and awake. These thoughts can be a subtle, barely detectable underlying thread. They might be wisps of thoughts; failure, unattractive, alone, weak. Instead of helping ourselves, these thoughts bring negative feelings and negative results.

Don't let your lack of self love limit how much you can love your children, your spouse and your friends. Be gentle and kind with the words you tell yourself. Trust yourself and treat yourself with self respect.

The Awakened Life

In contrast to an unconscious way of living, we are presented with yoga. Yoga opens a portal back to awareness and your inner self, reigniting that childhood essence of enthusiasm and joy. To be truly happy, we can choose to be a warrior for our own health and happiness, developing genuine compassion for ourselves as we reach to find our way to a life that really works for us.

Can we learn to tell ourselves a new story? Can we learn to embrace our imperfections and vulnerabilities? How do we begin?

Start by feeding your mind the positive thoughts that produce the results you want. This is the opposite of worry. Worry is like praying for what you don't want. Ask yourself, "What am I thinking about? What I don't want - or what I want? Am I building myself up or limiting myself by my beliefs?"

As we dedicate ourselves to the practices of yoga, we learn how to unravel untruths we've believed about ourselves and the world. These untruths have kept us bound long enough. It's time to take the journey toward an authentically meaningful life.

This journey to a meaningful life requires a willingness and a stillness that is uncommon in our hectic lives. Carlos Castaneda, best selling author of the classic book, *The Teachings of Don Juan: A Yaqui Way of Knowledge*, refers to this uncommon life as the life of a warrior. Castaneda says, "A warrior lives his life strategically."

Whether you've been doing yoga for years or never rolled out a yoga mat in your life, everything can shift for you. As you explore the path of yoga, you can heal your body and transform your life. Practicing self inquiry, meditation, focus and the poses will lead you back to where you began as a child with unbridled enthusiasm. Yoga can be your vehicle of change, taking you into your true core of unlimited inspiration to find greater happiness and freedom.

Create A New Story

Every yoga class gives us an opportunity to listen to our thoughts and hear what we are saying to ourselves, our "story." The final pose is always savasana, which means corpse pose. Things don't get much more still than death, and listening is the purpose of this pose. After moving our body through the physical practice, we are open, clear and receptive. In the stillness of corpse, we can hear what we tell ourselves.

Listening to the quiet, you can begin to hear your thoughts. What are the default thoughts that you revert to? Do they uplift you and inspire you? Or do they wear you down with worry? Maybe it's time to put to rest the habit of focusing on your faults and replace it with a focus on trusting your strengths.

This final pose is the perfect time to notice the thoughts we are feeding our mind and perhaps choose a different theme. We can begin telling ourselves, "I am strong. I do my best. I can trust myself and my inner guidance." Changing your thoughts will change the storyline of your days. Create a new story for yourself which is based on a deep trust in your own ability.

The power of this new story is immense. In this new story lies the influence and the ability for you to change your life.

You are exactly where you are today because of the work that you have already done. It has brought you to this point. This is your moment.

The tools and practices presented in the following chapters can be used whenever you need them. You can continue to explore them, going as deep as you want into a lifetime of learning. The exercises in the following chapters are simple but powerful, and can be the catalysts for lasting change. They work.

Enjoy a guided meditation to help you fully relax
in savasana, the final pose of practice, by visiting
www.CatherineMazurYoga.com/guidedrelaxation

Chapter Nine
Eight Steps To Bliss

*"The instant one begins to live like a warrior,
one is no longer ordinary."*

- Carlos Castaneda, *Journey to Ixtlan*

And Now Yoga

Little is known about the exact origins of yoga. Ordinary people who wanted to live extraordinary lives began to search for a system of health and happiness that was different from what they had been doing. They were looking for something that really worked for them.

This search revealed a profoundly modern discovery which anticipated quantum physics. The ancient yogis pointed out a subtle vibratory energy which now is recognized as the underlying connection between all things in the universe, the substratum of everything we know.

But where did this all begin?

The earliest forms of yoga have been speculated to date back to pre-vedic Indian traditions, but most likely developed around the fifth and sixth centuries BCE. Over the centuries, the yogic traditions have grown, morphed and shifted between philosophical, spiritual, energetic and physical practices.

Yoga gurus from India introduced yoga to the West. Soon afterwards, it became popular as a system of physical exercise across the Western world. This physical form of yoga is often called Hatha yoga, and is what most people consider to be the whole of yoga. However, it is so much more.

We can trace modern yoga to the sage, Patanjali, who lived somewhere around the second century BCE. The truth is that nobody really knows exactly when Patanjali lived. He's considered to be the father of modern yoga and somewhat of a Renaissance man, and is credited for developing and codifying yoga into eight powerful steps called Ashtanga yoga.

Even though it seems odd to us that so little is known about Patanjali, anonymity was typical of the great sages in ancient India. They recognized that their teaching was the outcome of a cooperative group effort that spanned several generations and refused to take credit for themselves.

Patanjali did not invent yoga. Yoga was already there and in various forms which he assimilated into the system. Perhaps he saw that yoga was getting too diversified and complex for anyone to understand in any meaningful way. So, he assimilated and included all aspects of the yoga of that current day into a certain format known as the yoga sutras.

The word sutra literally means thread or, in modern language, we can say it's like a formula. One thread leads to a whole train of thought or explanation. Patanjali began his short book of sutras with the following half sentence, "And now yoga."

Such a strange way to begin! It was almost as if he was saying if you're absorbed in thinking about anything trivial or material, it's not yet time for the serious study of true yoga. But if you've tasted everything in your life and you have realized that nothing is going to fulfill you ultimately, then it is time for yoga. In other words, if you come to a place where you feel nothing works and you don't have a clue about what it's all about - now yoga.

Actually, the yoga sutras aren't even really a book, they are more like a complex collection of tools arranged in a brilliant way, and in them we are introduced to the foundational building blocks of life changing yoga.

A Vibrational Universe

As the early yogis discovered- this is a vibrational universe. Everything down to the tiniest particle is vibrating. The brilliant Albert Einstein questioned the absolute "physical" solid nature of matter. This is because all matter is made up of tiny atomic and subatomic particles separated by relatively huge amounts of space compared to their size.

Gases have more spaces between particles then do solids because gas particles vibrate at a higher frequency. All matter consists of small particles, protons and neutrons, all held together by *energy* with relatively large distances between them.

Everything is composed mostly of space with particles vibrating in it. Every cell in our body is charged and vibrates at a different frequency. The denser the object, the more slowly its atoms vibrate. Interestingly, when a high frequency energy field is introduced to a low-frequency energy field, the lower frequency is drawn up to match a higher frequency.

All of our trillions of cells have a vibrational charge and even our thoughts carry an electric, vibrational charge. When we have a happy thought, it causes a high, light feeling vibration. A worry or fearful thought produces a heavy vibration which we feel as a dense, heavy, lower vibration. When we focus our thoughts on something that delights us, we raise our vibration and attract other things of similar vibration into our awareness and into our life.

Feelings are forms of energy vibrating at a lower or higher frequency. Love, gratitude and joy are high frequencies. Grief, anger and resentment are low frequencies energies.

These vibrational charges act like energy magnets to attract like vibrations to themselves. In recent years, much has been written and taught about this "law" which states that like attracts like. What you think about all day long is what you become. Thoughts create things. This is the essence of the Law of Attraction.

If you look closely within the ancient texts of Patanjali's yoga, you can find the seeds of the Law of Attraction outlined in the eight limbs, or eight steps.

The Eight Limbs

The eight limbs of yoga, as delineated in the yoga sutras, are steps we can take to shift our vibration to a higher state. From there, we can choose the thoughts and ideas that we want to experience in our life, things that bring us joy, empower us and delight us.

Your vibrational, focused thoughts act as a magnet to draw events, situations and similar manifestations into your life. Still powerful today, these ancient steps provide you with a practical way of living happily in the world while gradually moving your consciousness forward. This eight step system of yoga is the structure from which much of today's yoga has sprung, including vinyasa and hot yoga.

Because the Western world has emphasized the physical part of yoga, the other seven steps of yoga have been largely ignored. The average practitioner misses out on the deeper power of the practice which is the life changing purpose of the entire system of yoga.

Below are the eight limbs, or steps, to give us an introduction to the entire yoga process designed to work together as a whole.

We follow the steps as they take us inward through healing and awareness that ultimately brings us happiness and peace.

The Yamas, or social behaviors, are the most external of these eight limbs. These behaviors are universally accepted ethics such as truthfulness and nonviolence.

Niyamas, or personal behaviors, are the second limb. These dictate how we should focus our personal behaviors.

The Yamas include:

Ahimsa ~ Non-violence

Satya ~ Truthfulness

Asteya ~ Non-stealing

Brahmacharya ~ Non-excess

Aparigraha ~ Non-possessiveness

The Niyamas include:

Saucha ~ Purity

Santosha ~ Contentment

Tapas ~ Self-discipline

Svadhyaya ~ Self-study

Ishvara Pranidhana ~ Surrender

Together, these ten ethical precepts allow us to be at peace with ourselves, our family and our community. They guide us in how to conduct ourselves and then how to interact with others. It's about doing to others as you would want them to do to you. You know - the Golden Rule.

It all starts here because we are interconnected with each other and with everything in the universe. What we do to others, we truly do to ourselves. Everything affects everything. The principles set forth in the yamas and niyamas are high vibration energy principles. As we practice them we affect, not only our own vibrational field, but also the vibration of those around us and of the entire universal unified field.

Asana is the third limb, which includes the physical postures that most people associate with the word yoga. The asanas, or postures, keep our body flexible, strong and healthy. Although we are spiritual beings, we ARE on a human journey. Our human bodies are amazing instruments that need to be maintained to operate at their peak performance so we can best explore all the possibilities for personal creativity and happiness here on earth. The yoga poses also move energy in our body, releasing blocked and stuck patterns of holding, freeing us from emotional wounds and limiting beliefs.

Pranayama is the fourth limb. This is the practice of breath regulation, and begins to affect us on a more subtle level, beginning to purify the mind. Breath is an immediate and powerful tool to quiet the body and the mind. Besides being critical for cellular function, it carries a subtle energy into our bodies that changes our experience of life. Through breathing exercises, or pranayama, we manipulate our subtle energy to change the flow of thought, mood and ultimately behavior.

Pratyahara is the fifth limb and it brings us further inward by removing sense distractions from the mind. We train ourselves to look inward to produce the results we want, instead of looking at outward signs. This skill is essential to creating the kind of life that we want to live. We learn to cultivate a higher vibrational state and thought pattern to stay focused on our own desires for our life, based on our unique talents, gifts and essence. We begin to become masters of our own destiny, creating the results we desire by working from the inside out, rather than from the outside in. When we let the outside world define and direct us, it leads to unhappiness, limitation and fear.

Remember Harv? Harv learned to live his life from the inside out, doing what he loved without worrying about how he appeared to others. What freedom there is in this! Like Harv, many of us have lived most of our lives as a slave to how we think we are supposed to live. The following three steps, or limbs, help us to go inward so that we can know what our deepest desires really are and then live in a way that is authentic and fulfilling.

Dharana is first of three "inner" limbs of Patanjali's ashtanga yoga. The last three limbs all take place in one's consciousness. Dharana enables one to focus attention. This is the single most useful tool one can learn, the power of focused attention.

The mind is the greatest force in all of creation and as we train it to focus on the object of our desire, we summon universal powers of creation. This strong, single focus creates a strong vibrational pull. The previously mastered limbs, which are the practices of yoga asana, breathwork and meditation are all ways to teach ourselves to focus. Once we train the brain to focus, we have begun to unlock the secret to a calm mind, happy heart, and the ability to create the life experience that we desire.

Dhyana Dhyana is the seventh limb. It is the ability to maintain a sustained focus on a single object. This object can be a mantra, idea or attitude. In Part Two, we will continue to explore the power of the mind and discover that cultivating the ability to focus is the key to reprogramming the subconscious. This is the secret to obtaining the results and the change that you desire in your life.

Samadhi is the result of this sustained focus. It is the eighth and last limb. When we become so completely absorbed in the object of our meditation or focus that there is no perceived separation between the subject and object, we experience the bliss of being. In other words, we have tapped into the secret of the universe, and have learned the secret of the power to create. Here, on the leading edge of all creation, we use focus and desire to influence the ever expanding universe as it unfolds. Our maintained high frequency vibration raises any lower vibrations and attracts the essence of our focus, which leads to bliss. This is powerful and exciting stuff!

It is this Law of Attraction, as it is often referred to, that brings samadhi or bliss. We learn how, through the power of sustained focus, to draw the object of our focus into our experience. The resulting feeling is a sense of peace and empowerment which comes from unity and the realization that all is one. Our sustained focus creates our reality.

Want to learn more about using the Law of Attraction to consciously create a life that you love?

Visit **www.CatherineMazurYoga.com/resources**

PART TWO

THE MIND

*"If you have controlled your mind,
you have controlled everything."*

- Swami Satchidananda

Think!

Chapter Ten
The Path Of Knowledge

"You're ready to grow when you finally realize that the "I"
who is always talking inside will never be content.
It always has a problem with something."
- Michael A. Singer, *The Untethered Soul*

Connie had been coming to my 6am yoga class for a couple months, and one morning she came up to me after class with an interesting magazine article about meditation and the practice self awareness. That was the beginning of an ongoing conversation we had about self inquiry which we continued for a couple years.

After time, we both moved on, me to a different teaching schedule, and her to a new job. A few months ago I received an email from her with the following story:

So, in my new job in Torrey Pines, in the most beautiful place in the world in the open minded city of San Diego, I have a very large office that is off in the corner, away from everyone and I barely get any visitors.

The company has a lunchtime yoga program twice a week with a wonderful instructor. They spend a lot of money on Wellness programs including a session on Mindfulness from San Diego University. Their slogan is to help others live healthy lives.

What a wonderful place! I thought it would be perfect to take occasional short breaks to be able to meditate and do a little stretching and yoga - to release my back and clear my mind. In my secluded office space, I can close the blinds and lock the door for privacy while I stretch for a few minutes and then unlock and open for business, renewed and refreshed.

In the first month, the janitor busted in to dump the trash and caught me in a yoga pose on the floor. He said, "Oh, were you sleeping?" and, shocked at his intrusion, I just kind of mumbled something.

A little later, I was called into human resources for feedback about how I was fitting in. Apparently there had been complaints and said that I was caught "sleeping" in my office.

Having recently lost a job, I was frightened beyond belief that I was getting fired again.

I knew I needed to change the perception of my coworkers, so I shifted my behavior, including putting a small sign on my door while I was meditating. After a month or so, things smoothed out and I got a thumbs up from the HR department.

Shortly afterwards, I got a new boss and he said that my coworkers were offended by my sign. Although he said he is a meditator, it was the sign on my door that he found offensive.

I was struck by the apparent hypocrisy of the company and felt my coworkers were being arrogant and disrespectful.

There are many issues involved in this story, including policies, perceptions and beliefs, but what is interesting to me is not who is right or wrong, but rather, the following email that Connie sent me a few weeks later.

I wrote you a summary of what happened to me when I was meditating in my office. I've been thinking a lot about it and have concluded that it is I who has a lack of respect for those around me.

My thoughts are that I am not being aware of the attitudes of those around me and even look down on them because they aren't as "hip" or "enlightened" as I am. Wow, what a revelation! I am the one being arrogant and disrespectful to put a big sign on my door saying I'm meditating, not taking into consideration that they don't understand and probably have some discomfort about it.

I can be a bit of a snob, thinking I'm better than those around me - the books I read, the habits I have of yoga, meditation, writing. I want to be in an environment where it is accepted and so I push it, thinking that I can make them like it.

The Practice Begins In The Mind

Connie practiced self awareness to recognize the beliefs that she held which were causing her to suffer, and then she used that knowledge to practice understanding and compassion. She decided to take a step back from her current belief and examine it; this is the practice of self awareness.

The brain is a dynamic internal organ of intelligence. It is always busy calculating, analyzing, judging, and organizing information. Our brain's job is to generate thought and our challenge is to take a step back and examine our thoughts dispassionately and recognize that we are not the thoughts that our brain generates.

Yoga Stills The Mental Chatter

The second yoga sutra says, "Yoga stills the mind's chatter." Mental chatter or fluctuating thoughts, as some translate it, is the never ending commentary taking place inside our head.

"I hate this job. I should look for a new one. NO! You are secure here. I can do better. Oh come on, remember what happened last time you changed jobs? Don't be ridiculous."

Who's talking? Who's listening? Notice that the voice takes both sides of the conversation. It doesn't care which side it takes, just as long as it gets to keep up the mental chattering. It can drive us nuts.

Thoughts don't think, or judge themselves as good or bad. They can be accepted or rejected. They all have equal power to become reality. Practicing yoga, we learn to breathe and observe. We observe how our body feels and we observe the commentary that our inner thoughts obsess about.

In yoga class, our thoughts may ridicule our efforts and then take us off onto some fantasy tangent. "This is hard. Why didn't I eat something first? I wonder what I will make for dinner?"

I forgot to buy eggs. What did the teacher just say? I'll follow that girl in front of me, she's really good. Oh, I like this pose…. I bet she thinks she's a star. Don't judge!"

We all have wild monkey minds, jumping around from branch to branch. To help us with this, a large part of the yoga writings are about how to control our mentality. How? Begin with self study and taking a step back from this incessant brain chatter to view it objectively.

When we begin to control our mentality and recognize that we are the thinker of these random thoughts, we begin to resist identifying so strongly with our thoughts themselves. Then we can begin to see ourselves as the witness of our thoughts and thoughts for what they are; random wisps in our electronic circuitry that we can entertain or laugh at.

Thoughts are energy and energy can be converted into matter. This is why controlling our mentality is so critically important.

Choose your thoughts! Turn off the power to thoughts that make you feel bad. Amp up the volume of your positive thoughts.

If we are constantly thinking about what we don't want, eventually we will see it show up in some form in our lives. Don't spend your time and energy there. Instead, dream more! Create thoughts that thrill you and watch how your life changes.

Brain Vs Mind

No one has ever seen the mind. Autopsies reveal the organs in the body including the brain, but the mind cannot be seen. It can only be experienced. Mind is that part of us that yogis call the witness or atman. It is the unchanging part of us that can take a step back and watch our thoughts. The mind is not located in any particular part of our bodies, rather it is in every cell within us. The mind is universal intelligence.

It's with our mind that we create the intention to care for our brain. We can use our brain, molding in it and learning to shape our thoughts. We can teach ourselves how to think, consciously choosing the thoughts that will bring us happiness and success.

When we see that the brain is really just an organ of the body, like the heart or lungs, we can begin to dissociate with the thinking process and can question our thoughts as separate from who we are. We are not our thoughts, but rather we are the consciousness behind the thoughts.

The heart's job is to pump blood through our body, just as the lungs job is to continually exchange oxygen and carbon dioxide. Our stomachs secrete digestive juices and our liver detoxes our blood. These are the functions of the innately intelligent organs within our body. They perform these functions on their own, without needing any conscious thought directing them to do so.

And so, as we take a closer look, we can recognize that the brain's job is to think. Analyzing, passing judgements, imagining dangers - real or not, are among the frequent memos it sends us. It does this constantly.

To keep us safe from dangers, the brain is hyper alert, tossing up every possible scenario that could happen. It indiscriminately serves up everything from fear of driving off the road unexpectedly to dropping the baby. These thoughts can be extremely unnerving when we believe that we ARE our thoughts.

Because many of our brain's warnings, suggestions, and fears are ridiculous, we can use them to examine the thinking process and take a step back from it all. We may not have control over what randomly pops into our brain, but we do have the choice as to whether we accept or reject those thoughts. When we realize that we have the option to utterly reject some of our thoughts and exercise control over what we choose to focus upon, we begin to make a huge stride towards change.

Who Are You?

As we become adept at recognizing that we are not our thoughts, we realize that there is a separation between our thoughts and our actual self.

We understand this when we remember ourselves as a five year old, a teen or as a young adult. We are the same self, but the thoughts that we think today are not the thoughts of a five-year-old or a teen. Thank goodness for that!

We are the same person, although we've obviously changed over the years, and so naturally our thoughts are different; therefore, we can say that we are not our thoughts.

We notice this when we sit down to meditate or quiet our thoughts. Sometimes we just want to still our racing mind's intense activity. As soon as we settle in and try to focus on relaxing and just stop thinking, the brain begins to serve up its incessant chatter. Our minds wander off in one direction or another, usually reworking whatever problems we are currently wrestling with. Eventually, we wake up and realize that we are far from having a quiet mind and once again try to quiet our thoughts. Before long, we find ourselves off following the very same tangent, or a new worry or problem.

Who is it that recognizes we've wandered off? And who is it that decides to again try to drop the thought? It's as if there are two of us inside; one who wanders off and one who says, "Whoa, wait a minute, come back here!"

Yoga tradition teaches that the one who sees is the witness. This witness within us is known as the soul, or atman, and is our innermost essence. Atman is unchanging and eternal and is sometimes referred to as the observer or the mind. This part of us is always at peace. When we find ourselves disturbed, confused, or worried we are identifying with the ego or brain and have moved away from our center.

Create A Perfect Life

Everything we see around us that is man-made began as a thought. Every gadget in our kitchen drawers was first an idea in someone's brain. The most basic inventions, like the wheel, to the high tech computerized cars that sit upon them - all began as thoughts before they become a reality.

Our thoughts have tremendous power. They create our life experience, not only physical inventions, but also the mental and emotional experiences of our life. Our thoughts also create our degree of financial success, the quality of our relationships and our "luck."

Thoughts in the brain have a vibrational quality. The tight network of nerve cells in our brain generate an electrical field which can be detected by common medical equipment. Our internal electric field is governed by the same laws as the rest of the universe's electromagnetic spectrum. Thoughts are formed in this field and can be measured, showing that they are truly energy, just like everything else.

Quantum Physics And Mother Teresa

Leading-edge research in the field of quantum physics has shown that the process of thinking actually causes molecule movement, which creates an energetic wave, causing a reaction. A thought wave has the power to attract and repel, just as all phenomena in the electromagnetic spectrum attracts and repels.

The implication is that everything is interconnected, and so what happens in the field if the mind has a snowball effect out beyond the mind. Remember the butterfly wing theory? Any movement, anywhere, becomes a virtual wave which puts molecules in motion. These moving molecules affect the molecules around them causing a larger wave. Thought wave molecules become an essential element in the process of creation.

As we consciously choose the thoughts we think, we can affect the environment around us through this theory of entanglement. Our level of thought consciousness determines our reality. The higher vibration of the thoughts we have, the higher the level of our consciousness.

Mother Teresa knew the power of words and the power of thought. When asked if she was against war she replied, "I'm not against war, I'm for peace." She focused thought energy on what she wanted and stated it in the positive without giving any thought to the negative. She knew the secret to the most powerful way to bring change in the world - thinking high vibrational, positive thoughts.

Mother Teresa was right, of course.

Believe In Yourself

Start here. This practice is like giving yourself a hug. It is like being with your bestfriend, someone who really, really loves you unconditionally. Believe in your dreams, believe in your abilities and talents.

Avoid comparing yourself to anyone else. There will always be someone more successful and there will always be someone less successful. They don't matter. This is all about you.

Wake up each morning and remind yourself that you are doing the best you can and that you are an amazing person. If you do this simple practice throughout the day, you will immediately feel better.

In the following chapters as we explore Jnana yoga, the path of knowledge, you will learn some powerful tools to help you gain confidence and clarity for your life. Each practice is powerful on its own. Combined, they are life changing.

For more specific ways to raise your vibration
and live in a positive state, go to
www.CatherineMazurYoga.com/vibration

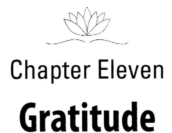

Chapter Eleven
Gratitude

"The further I wake into this life,
the more I realize that God is everywhere and
the extraordinary is waiting quietly
beneath the skin of all that is ordinary."
- Mark Nepo, *The Book of Awakening*

Gratitude

Very early one morning, my daughter walked into the kitchen took a piece of paper and began writing with intense focus. "What are you doing?" I asked.

"Mom, I just had the most amazing dream. I'm writing a note to myself to remember the message in the dream."

We had been sharing our dreams with each other for years; ever since I read about a tribe that ritually shared their dreams every morning in a community dream circle. This is not to be confused with creamsicle, the ice cream treat, but as it turns out, it's just as yummy and rewarding because there was virtually no illness or depression experienced by the members of this tribe.

"Tell me!" I was excited to hear the important message of her dream.

"I dreamt I was in the large auditorium filled with people. They were there to honor exceptional women and I was one of them!

The first woman was an internationally acclaimed author of seven New York Times bestselling books. She had changed countless people's lives through her writing. She accepted her award and when she stepped down from the podium, everyone applauded.

The next woman to speak on stage had written, directed and produced ten blockbuster films. Her accomplishments were exceptional, especially for a woman in that industry. When she accepted her award, people clapped and cheered.

I was called up to the stage next. I was so excited because I was so proud of my life, I felt good about what I had achieved. I stood behind the podium and this is what I said. She handed me the post it note on which she had written,

"I have lived an extraordinary ordinary life." We looked at each other and laughed because we knew it was both absurdly simple and supremely difficult.

When we live each day with gratitude, the ordinary becomes extraordinary. It is true that the extraordinary waits quietly beneath the skin of all that is ordinary and that we just need to look for it.

And when we make the choice to shift to a place of gratitude we open new pathways in our brain. Our brains actually change. In the same way that we strengthen our muscles when we exercise, we can train our brains.

Grateful thoughts are like little messengers that transmit positive energy throughout our entire bodies. The more we practice thoughts of gratitude, the more these pathways open up. And the more this positive energy flows, the more it strengthens our very being.

Gratitude is the secret to living a life filled with love. Love is the highest emotion and the highest vibrational state we can experience. Gratitude is a doorway that brings us into that vibration. When we're feeling grateful, our hearts feel light and open to love. Feeling gratitude, we instantly feel happier and appreciate everything and everyone who's in front of us.

Get quiet and see if you can sense the extraordinary beneath your everyday life. It will fill you with wonder, gratitude and love.

Action Steps

- Take one minute of quiet time every morning and evening
- Start a gratitude journal
- Begin your day by creating a mental "blessings list"

The extraordinary doesn't push to the forefront, it waits quietly to be discovered. As we practice gratitude, we realize how profoundly wondrous our ordinary life is.

As you begin to cultivate an attitude of expectation, every day you can experience something new. A wrong turn can lead to the discovery of a secluded park. A new yoga class might lead to the discovery of a pose you've never done before. The truth is that we really don't know what a day can bring. Unexpected discoveries and delights are all around us - we just need to open our eyes and ears and hearts.

For how to create a gratitude practice that can change your daily experience of life visit
www.CatherineMazurYoga.com/gratitudejournal

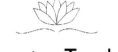

Chapter Twelve

Intentions and Affirmations

*"Things which matter most must never be
at the mercy of things which matter least."*
- Goethe

Tony's Story

*When Tony was a teenager, his parents went through a divorce and his
mom thought he was siding with his dad, so she kicked him out of the
house. On Christmas eve.*

*He had to figure out how to survive. He was seventeen years old,
still finishing high school and working as a janitor, doing the night
shift. He would take a couple buses to get to work, work really
hard, getting done around 1:30 in the morning and then jump
on the late night bus to start the long journey home to get to
school in the morning.*

*One night, he went out after his work was finished to wait for
the bus. He waited and waited, but it never came. He knew he hadn't
missed it because he couldn't afford to miss it. An hour, two hours, went*

by, and finally some guy came by and asked him what he was doing. "I'm waiting for the bus."

The guy told him that there was a bus strike. Tony had no one to call for a ride home, his friends didn't have cars, so he decided he didn't have any other option and began walking. As he walked, he realized that he would never get home in time at this rate. Then something inside him got very intense and he just snapped. Something inside told him, "You're going to find the way!" And he began to jog. He had never run more than a couple miles in his life.

He began an incantation as he ran. With every stride he said, "Every day in every way I'm getting stronger and stronger. Every day in every way I'm getting healthier and healthier!"

He ran for 12 miles that night. At the end of that run, he never felt stronger in his entire life. He felt as though he could storm through anything. Nothing was going to stop him.

This created a whole new momentum in his life that has continued to this day. It's almost 30 years later and Tony has taken the message of the power of an intention, he calls it an incantation, around the world. His message has impacted hundreds of thousands of people worldwide, from ordinary people like you and me to world leaders.

Maybe you have heard him speak, or have his cds. Tony Robbins is still changing lives today, teaching what he learned for himself; the power of a positive mentality and a strongly stated intention.

Your Internal Gps

Once you have connected to the energy of gratitude and belief in yourself, you are in the right frame of mind to create an intention.

An intention is a commitment to yourself. It acts like a road map for us. If we know we want to get to Santa Fe from San Diego, we need a map. Without a map, we would just head in the general direction and after many, many detours and turnarounds we would get closer by trial and error. We might get so lost that we decide to give up, turn around and head back. Eventually we would get there, but it would have been so much easier and a lot less frustrating if we had a map.

Intention is the map for our life. It is our plan to guide us efficiently towards our goals. First, we need to get clarity about what we really want. If we don't know what we want, how will we know what direction to go? How will we recognise it when we've arrived?

In every area of life, you will benefit from the help of a map. Intentions can be set for your day, for your business, and for your life. Even in a yoga class, it is common for the teacher to suggest the students set an intention for the hour.

As you get very clear, laser focused, on what you are looking for and desire for yourself, your intentions will help you move confidently in the right direction. The reward of a strong, clear intention is a strong clear direction for your day and your life.

Here are some tips to get you started to create an effective intention.

Action Steps

- **Imagine it.** The first step is to get really clear on what you want. There is a limitless quantum field of possibilities for creating anything and everything you want. An effective intention is always what you are looking for, not what you hope to avoid or change. So, be careful to state it in the positive. For example, "I want to feel energized and alive" rather than, "I'm not so exhausted all the time." "I find gratitude and joy at work" instead of "I'm not irritated by people today." You get the idea.

- **Feel it.** See it, imagine it. What would it feel like? This puts the energy in motion. Don't skip this step. Even if you take just 30 seconds - really tap into the feeling, letting it saturate your body and soul. (Magic here... I'm just sayin')
- **Write it.** Your results will be assured and amplified if you write it down and/or communicate it to someone. Especially for your bigger life intentions. Journaling is a form of manifestation; words on paper. This brings it into the material realm.
- **Share it.** Share your intention with a person who is safe, who supports you and will anchor your intention. It will also help to hold you accountable and give you an ally.

The field of possibilities is a vast, unlimited source. Every outcome, every blessing, and every option is valid in this field. Our opportunity is to choose what we want from this vast field. Once we have a desire, it is this setting of our intention that officially begins the creation process. So begin now, set an intention that feels exciting and follow with the other steps above.

Remember the universal Law of Attraction states like draws like. This law is as real as the law of gravity. Just like our yoga, the more we practice setting intentions for everything in our life, the easier it becomes to do. As we exercise our intention habit, the Law of Attraction will continue to surprise and delight us.

Let your intentions pave the way for your growth and success.

Affirmations

Affirmations are positive statements describing a desired situation, which are often repeated until they get impressed on the subconscious mind. Using affirmations is an important tool for creating a strong mentality and creating the desired results in your life.

Affirmations work on a couple different levels.

Our subconscious mind drives our behavior, not our conscious intentions. How many times have you tried over and over to change a habit or behavior and just can't do it? This is because your subconscious is running a different program that will ultimately drive your behavior, not your conscious willpower or intent.

You need to reprogram your subconscious mind. Affirmations will work to change your behavior because repetition is key to impressing the thought upon subconscious mind, transforming it into a belief.

Affirmations are a proven method for self-improvement because they actually rewire our brains. This process pushes the subconscious mind to take action to make the positive statement a reality.

To learn the exact steps to create daily affirmations that work like magic to take your life to a whole new level, visit
www.CatherineMazurYoga.com/affirmations

Chapter Thirteen

Visualization And Changing The Channel

"You live in a vibrational universe."
- Abraham-Hicks

*R*eza was tired of dating the wrong women. He was ready to settle down with the perfect woman and was frustrated that he wasn't able to find her. His friend Veronica advised him to begin picturing this perfect lady every morning and every night. "Picture every detail, her voice, her walk, her eyes, and do this daily for three months solid and she'll show up," she said. "That's how I met my fiance, Dave." Reza decided to give it a try, even if it was just a fun experiment because he had nothing to lose. Somewhere around the third month into his daily perfect woman visualization practice, he was at work and felt someone brush by him. He got an uncanny sensation as he heard a voice at the end of the counter and looked up to see his dream girl. Coincidence? Reza doesn't think so. They were married 9 months later.

Visualization

Visualization is a mental technique that uses the imagination to manifest goals and dreams. It is one more layer that you can use to control your mentality and use your brain to create what you want in life. When you know how to use creative visualization effectively it will supercharge your other practices of intention setting and affirmations. When you can visualize yourself as the ocean rather than the drop, your possibilities expand exponentially.

Creative visualization is the practice of seeking to affect the outer world by using the brain's ability to see a mental picture in the mind. It is a way to look at things differently and in doing so, everything changes. And because we think in images, the stronger the image, the more powerful its effect on our subconscious.

By visualizing a certain event, situation or object you can actually attract it into your life. It's a process similar to daydreaming. If you want to attract something different into your life, change the pictures in your head. By changing your thoughts and mental images, you change your reality. You're not using any kind of magic, simply the natural powers and laws that everyone possesses. It's a basic technique frequently used by athletes to enhance their performance.

This sounds like "new age" stuff, but it's been recognized as a technique for manifestation for a long, long time. In the early 1900s, Wallace Wattles wrote *The Science of Getting Rich*. In it, he advocates creative visualization as the main technique for realizing one's goal based on a practice that stems from an ancient Hindu theory of the universe described in the book.

Nothing New Under The Sun

In the yoga system of Patanjali, which has been around for centuries, creative visualization is used in the sixth and seventh steps of his eight limb system. **Dharana** refers to cultivating focused attention and **dhyana** is the practice of maintaining one's acute focus on a single object. Visualization is heightened in the brain when the focus is maintained with closed eyes.

Although Patanjali didn't include closing the eyes as part of the process, focus can include looking at an object, contemplating a sutra, or visualizing a desired outcome.

Reza is in good company in his visualization practice because celebrities like Oprah Winfrey, Bill Gates, Tiger Woods, Will Smith, Arnold Schwarzenegger, Anthony Robbins and Jim Carrey use visualization to overcome challenges and claim it plays a significant role in their success.

Violet's 5 Channels

Visualization is a powerful tool to change the direction of your life. It works by changing your state. To change your life, change your state. First you need to determine what triggers you to drop from a high vibration, happy state into a low vibration or emotion.

Violet Rainwater, sales coach and creator of Bizasana, has created a process called the mindmap. The mindmap represents the human mind broken down into five channels; the higher channels representing higher regions of the mind, and the lower channels representing the lower. Each channel represents a certain mindset and the results associated with it.

These mindsets, or channels, are more than just thoughts or moods. They are actually a mindset vibration which creates a wave that produces a particular feeling, just as turning to a specific radio channel, or airwave, will tune into a specific station. These waves correlate to Violet's five channels and the resulting attitudes and behaviors.

Her very effective process begins by determining what channel you are on when you first wake up in the morning. From that baseline, you notice when your channel changes and what triggered the change. Here are the channels.

- **Channel 5** is the highest channel. When we're tuned into channel 5, we're at the top of our game. We feel enthusiastic, inspired, and passionate. This state is that "top of the world" feeling in which we feel empowered, compassionate, grateful, and filled with love. It is an exceptional day! We have those rare days when we awaken with this feeling, and when we continue to stay tuned to this high channel it becomes a stellar day.

- **Channel 4** is also a high vibrational channel. This is a very peaceful state. It's important to linger here every day through breathwork, meditation, yoga, or even napping! Channel 4 recharges you so that you can move through your day with ease and grace; tranquil but enthused. When we're tuned into channel 4, life is good and we feel clear, productive, and happy.

  The results of being in these higher channels are innovation, cooperation, productivity, focus, vision, accountability, creativity, and trust.

- **Channel 3** is most people's default zone. Our day is "fine" and we are feeling "okay." We are going through the motions, but not feeling particularly charged or energized.

- **Channel 2** is the channel that we are tuned into when we feel frustration, doubt, disappointment, guilt, worry, discouragement, or pessimism. Most of us dip down into this channel 2 vibration on a regular basis.

- **Channel 1** is the lowest frequency and one that we seldom, if ever visit. Here we feel rage, depression, fear, powerlessness, and unworthiness.

The results we get when we are tuned into these three lower channels are mediocre to dismal. Morale is low, as is our performance. We fall into blame, small thinking, gossip, and disrespect.

Action Step

There is a simple solution to change your channel so that you can stay inspired and enthusiastic. By learning how to tune in to your "triggers" and then turn it around, you can avoid dipping into discouragement and worry.

Learn 3 simple steps to change your channel
www.CatherineMazurYoga.com/channelchanging

Chapter Fourteen
Big Bad Beliefs

*"One does not become enlightened
by imagining figures of light, but
by making the darkness conscious."*

- Carl Jung

Byron's Big Assumption

Byron Katie tells the story about one day walking into the ladies room in a restaurant and meeting a woman coming out of the stall. They smiled and as the woman washed her hands, she began to sing. Katie thought it was a lovely voice. Going into the stall, she noticed that the toilet seat was dripping wet. She thought, "How rude! And how did she manage to pee all over the seat?" Then it came to her that "she" was a man, a transvestite, singing falsetto in the women's restroom! As she cleaned the toilet seat, she fumed and thought about everything she would like to say to "him." Then she flushed the toilet and the water shot up out of the bowl and flooded the seat. She stood there laughing at herself and her fantastical story based on pure assumption.

"Never assume anything" is one of the "Agreements" from Miguel Ruiz's classic book, *The Four Agreements*, and it's a real eye opener. We make assumptions all day long without ever realizing it. We assume we should be smarter, thinner, richer, that traffic should move faster. We assume we should be able to eat things that aren't supporting our body, sleep for four hours and be able to function optimally. We assume our partner knows what we want and is just withholding it, we assume the car next to us is honking at us and the driver is a jerk (when it's not and she isn't).

Think of something that is painful and more often than not, we have created a belief that is more of an assumption than a fact.

Question Your Stories

Take something that is bothering you, causing you to suffer in some way, and ask yourself what belief you have underneath that is the source of your pain. There IS a belief that is the basis of your personal discomfort, whether your discomfort is anger, fear or sadness.

Then take that belief and get curious about it. Pull it to pieces. Inquire into what lies at the bottom of your belief that is causing you pain. Then ask yourself, "Is this really true? Can I absolutely know that it is true?"

How often do you assume to know what someone else is thinking just by the look on their face? Oh yes, you are very sure about it. But can you absolutely know what they are thinking? Have you ever asked them and been dead wrong?

All day long we assume things that simply are not true. We assume life should be this way or that way; when it's not, we suffer. We assume people should be kind and life should be fair. We spend a great deal of time assuming people are judging us, when the truth is, everyone is in their own head anyways.

All these assumptions can drive us crazy and make us suffer needlessly. Our assumptions about other people and what they think take up vast quantities of our daily energy.

The solution to this predicament is to question your conclusions and to never assume anything. When we become tuned in enough to listen to our own thoughts and question them, we will see just how much of what we think during the day is an assumption.

It is insane to continue the practice of believing things that we simply don't know are absolutely true, especially since they cause us to suffer.

These stories, or assumptions about what is real, can be about the past, present or future. They can be about what things should be or could be. They are about the untested, uninvestigated theories we have.

ACTION STEPS

- **Catch it.** Notice when a strong or uncomfortable emotion arises in you.

- **Question it.** Begin to question your thoughts when you feel upset or uncomfortable. Ask yourself if you are making an assumption about something. How much of your world is made up of untrue stories?

- **Change it!** Use the tools in this book or found on my website to help you catch yourself in the act of assuming, question your conclusions, and change your habits.

For a powerful process to free yourself from assumptions and limiting beliefs, visit my website
www.CatherineMazurYoga.com/assumptions

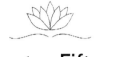

Chapter Fifteen
The Answers Within

*"I have something inside of me that trumps
everything that goes on outside of me."*
- Wayne Dyer

The human brain contains more than 100 billion neurons, more connections than there are stars in the universe. And each of these neurons can have 1 million connections each. That's a lot of activity.

All of that activity can become overwhelming considering the amount of data our brains receive throughout the day. Sorting and organizing this data happens in a micro second, and much of the data is never consciously perceived or we would be in information overload. We need a mental recess.

Quiet Time

If you read the biographies of great men and women, you will find that they all practiced some form of quiet time and daily designated time to take a step back to contemplate alone in stillness. Quiet time is different than the practice of meditation.

The practice of taking quiet time every day is simply taking time to give your brain a rest and to find the answers within.

This habit just might be the most important time of your day, the time when you escape from all the craziness of your schedule to sit somewhere just to contemplate. To unplug from all external stimuli and take time to just BE with yourself connects you to your inner resources. This quiet time and it's benefits are greatly magnified if you take it in nature.

A walk in the woods, a stroll on the beach, or even a chair pulled up to window to look upon a tree or garden will calm your soul and help you gain greater clarity. This connection with nature inspires us and keeps us present in the moment. It wakes us up to the larger reality of life. Our problems don't loom as largely when we are gazing at mountains and vast blue sky.

YOUR TRUSTED SOURCE

Quiet time is your opportunity to connect with your trusted source for guidance and inspiration. Your trusted source is something or someone whom you look to for the answers to such questions as, "What is right for me?" or "What is my purpose in life?" What in your universe knows the answer to your questions?

According to Tim Kelley, author of *True Purpose*, there are three basic types of trusted sources: internal, universal and personal.

An internal trusted source is exactly that. You consider this as some part of yourself. Some people refer to this as the soul or spirit, the witness or their higher self. It is something that you believe is present deep inside you, guiding you in some way even if you don't have a name for it. Consider for yourself if you feel you have an internal trusted source, or higher self.

A universal trusted source is something divine and outside of yourself. This source falls in the category of God or the universe.

It is an all powerful, all encompassing source that you believe is universal and available to everyone. Do you have a universal trusted source who you look to for answers to your deepest questions or prayers?

A personal trusted source could be a special guide, or loved one, an enlightened being or guardian angel who watches over you and guides you. It could be your grandma who is no longer alive but still feels present, looking over your shoulder making sure you're okay.

WISE CHOICES

If you are at a crossroad in your life or are facing a decision that you are struggling to make, these two practices will be a lighthouse guiding you onto the right course. To access the answers within begin the practice of daily quiet time and looking to your trusted source for guidance.

For help with accessing your deepest wisdom
so that you can find your answers visit
www.CatherineMazurYoga.com/theanswerswithin

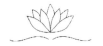

Chapter Sixteen
Enlightened Choices

"Between stimulus and response there is a space.
In that space lies our freedom and power to choose our response.
In our response lies our growth and freedom."
- Viktor Frankl

Rebecca's Story

Day 1

The day I filed for divorce, I decided my life wasn't over. It had just begun. So, I set out to travel this world.

I felt if I truly wanted to experience Rebecca, I needed to travel alone. I had been programmed as an infant, and throughout my life, to take care of the needs of others first. This journey was about me choosing me.

My metamorphosis started in the sludge of pain, sorrow and grief over my broken life. I was flattened by the thought of being 36, single and childless. Ironically, it was this part of my story that became the pivotal point of who I am today. Why? Because that was the day I chose me for the first time in my life. I committed to myself that I would take whatever time it took to heal the most important relationship in my life; my love affair with myself was to be rekindled.

So, I chose to travel with me, myself and I around the world. Over a year's time, I backpacked through Europe: Germany, Prague, Venice, and Rome. Then, a year later I backpacked throughout Bali, including the Gili Islands.

Talk about being vulnerable. And I don't mean to the dark alleys or "suspicious" foreigners. That is avoidable. I promise.

You really get to take a look inward when you are the only one around to talk to. And that was my mission. Who am I? What do I want? Which way do I want to go? Traveling alone forced these decisions to be made, and decision-making isn't my strong suit. There's no one to follow when you're travelling solo. Yes, some of my decisions were wonderful, yet came with tremendous challenges, obstacles, pain and opportunities for growth.

For example: I jump on my scooter right out the gate in Bali. Everyone warned me to be careful of the scooters and roads in Bali. "Shit, I got this, people!" I said. So, I hop on and punch it. Giving it too much gas, I couldn't turn. I drove straight across a busy road and crashed in a field.

Day 946

Who wants to spend 946 days working diligently on themselves? Let alone 946 days of ups, downs, turns and blocks? But as it turns out, 946 days in a land of loving yourself first isn't a bad place to be. No matter what it looks like.

Since Day 1, I have ventured out of my comfort zone. It began with my decision to leave an emotionally abusive marriage, which took the courage of a true warrior. It's scary as hell to leave something you know and are comfortable with no matter how unhealthy it is for your soul.

A true warrior is one who is able to be courageous and strong in their vulnerability. I found the warrior princess within as I allowed myself to push through my shame and guilt of a "failed" marriage and move into a space of authentically grasping what I desired: peace within.

During these 946 days of metamorphosis, my love for yoga increased. As I practiced throughout the world, I recognized one true theme: This space on my mat is where I truly connect to the inner Rebecca within. This space that I long for is created through my breath and when truly connecting to self. Which, for me, happens directly on my mat. I am deserving of this time and space. I put myself first by choosing to breathe with intention and fluidity.

In March of 2014, I took on the challenge of writing my blog: Still Playin' With It. This is another personal and highly vulnerable experience. Put your words and personal experiences out to the entire WORLD?! Yes, please. Sign me up. The true warrior princess emerges through her inner battles. The inner battles bring bravery and victories!

Today, day 947, I celebrate the victories in my life. I celebrate me. I celebrate me choosing me. I celebrate being Rebecca: a modern day Warrior Poet.

Every day you make choices that ultimately steer your life in one direction or another. Your choices should be based upon your values.

Your values are the ideas and things that you believe are important for the way you live and work. They determine your priorities and are the measure you use to decide if your life is turning out the way you wanted it to.

When the things you do and the way you behave match your values, life is usually good. But when they don't, that's when things feel wrong and can become a source of unhappiness. Making a conscious effort to identify your values is important in decision-making and answering your right questions.

Defining Your Values

A good place to begin is to identify the times when you were the happiest, when you were the most proud, and when you were the most fulfilled and satisfied. This will get you started in identifying what is most important to you in life.

This values exercise is a tough but enlightening process that will establish clear priorities for you. In your process, carefully analyze if these values are truly your own or if they are the voices of your parents, mentors, or upbringing. Stay anchored in the life values that bring personal meaning to you.

Taking a close look at your values is the starting point. Look over the list below, which are 20 of the 300 values I've listed on my website. They will help to get you thinking about exactly what is important to you.

Creativity	Honesty	Enjoyment
Compassion	Security	Tolerance
Generosity	Faith	Efficiency
Connection	Fitness	Mastery
Growth	Positivity	Decisiveness
Happiness	Loyalty	Prosperity
Health	Order	

Remember, as you carefully examine your values, you will refer to them as you make your daily choices. With your choices, you create your future. You are where you are today because of all the choices you've made in the past. Rather than using this as an excuse to fail or to berate yourself, use this knowledge as an inspiration to make better choices from today going forward. Change your life, one choice at a time.

Questions That Clarify

To find your answers, you need to ask certain questions of yourself. Prepare a list of compelling life questions based on your values. These questions will guide you and support you in making the right choices.

The Right Questions, Debbie Ford's innovative book on making better decisions for life, is an excellent resource to help you formulate your own questions. Her questions are deceptively simple but incredibly powerful and can be used in any situation or at any crossroads.

The following questions will illuminate the path before you and bring clarity:

- Will this choice add to my life force, or will it rob me of my energy?
- Am I standing in my power, or am I trying to please another?
- Will this choice propel me toward an inspiring future, or will it keep me stuck in the past?

Action Steps

- **Compose.** Compose a list of your values using the processes above.
- **Create.** Create your own right questions. Your questions should be based on your personal values balanced with your vision of your higher purpose in life. If you really want to change your life, you must make new choices. Your questions should wake you up and give you the power you need to change the direction of your life.
- **Consider.** Make a wish list for all the things you want in your life. Be honest, no one will see this but you. Pose your questions to each of the things on your wish list to see how they line up with your values. This is an illuminating exercise which causes you to look for the deeper value beneath the outer wanting.

To help you with the above action steps I've created a list of 300 values to download and begin to consciously create your future starting today.

www.CatherineMazurYoga.com/300values

PART THREE

THE BODY

*"If a person advances confidently
in the direction of their dreams,
and endeavors to live the life they've imagined,
they will meet unexpected success in common hours."*
- Henry David Thoreau

Move!

Chapter Seventeen
The Path Of Action

"I am rooted, but I flow."
- Virginia Woolf

The healing process of yoga is a holistic one. The four paths are a complete healing system of mind, body, soul and spirit. Here in Karma yoga, the path of action, you will learn about actions, including healing your body, being proactive about your health, and consciously choosing how you take action in the world, including in your relationships and community.

In the path of action, we explore all things karma. Karma yoga is the path of the warrior. Committed to action and results, the person who practices karma yoga knows the difference between knowing and doing. Knowledge must lead to action because words without deeds mean nothing.

Taking a very broad look at the path of action will include learning about all the principles of karma yoga. They are right action, right attitude, right speech, and right motive. That covers a lot!

Most of us are familiar with the term "karma" as something that will happen to us if we don't follow the golden rule. Although not entirely correct, it is not too far from the truth.

Remember Val's story and how we learned that everything is interrelated? Physical pain, emotional pain and mental pain are usually bound together in mysterious ways. What we sow, we reap, and we need to explore every action and reaction that we have. We need to learn how to take care of our bodies, hearts and minds, so we can find a balance that keeps us happy and healthy and allows the energy that flows through us to continue to flow. Stuck energy can be the source of much suffering.

Stuck energy can be a major source of pain in our body and hurt in our heart. It is usually the cause of the habitual patterns we repeat over and over, keeping us stuck in disfunction.

In the following chapters, you will learn physical yoga poses to heal your body. You will also learn the interrelated actions of being proactive in all areas of your health.

Right Action. Right Attitude. Right Speech. Right Motives.

For a list of great charitable organizations to practice the spirit of right action visit **www.CatherineMazurYoga.com/charities**

Chapter Eighteen
Knowing Vs Doing

"As the mind, so the man.
Bondage and liberation are in your own mind.
If you consider yourself bound, you are bound.
If you consider yourself liberated, you are liberated.
Things outside neither bind nor liberate you,
only your attitude towards them does that."

- Patanjali, *The Yoga Sutras*

We usually know the right things to do, like avoiding sugar, eating greens, getting eight hours of sleep, regular exercise and yoga; but the problem is - we don't do them.

There is a huge difference between knowing and doing.

We know what to do, but we don't do it - WHY?

When we know what to do and don't do it, there is gap between our conscious mind and subconscious mind. We get an idea, make a plan, decide to implement the plan, but then we don't follow through. This is crazy. Where is the disconnect between knowing what to do and doing it? Obviously, some larger part of us doesn't agree with the plan and won't follow through, no matter how sincerely we plan.

The problem is that our subconscious mind has another deeper agenda, and it sabotages our intentions. When we know what we want and what we need to do, but don't do it, we feel stuck. And frustrated. And sometimes defeated and depressed. When we feel as if we are always struggling with ourselves and trying but aren't getting the results that we are looking for, we need look deeper.

Actually, the subconscious mind is nothing but neural pathways that have been established in your brain as a result of your past beliefs and conditioning. Limiting beliefs, negative conditioning and misguided perceptions that you took to be true (can you absolutely KNOW?) caused strong patterns of thought to become subconscious.

These pathways are real and as strong as ropes that can hold you where you no longer want to be. A lot of times you realize certain truths and gain clarity, but are frustrated that your brain is not able to sync up with this understanding. We need to reprogram our subconscious. How do we do that? What is the solution?

4 Steps To Reprogram Your Brain

Look at some area of your life where you're not getting results you want. Ask yourself what would be the opposite of what you are getting? What would it be like, feel like, look like? Maybe you would be more calm, feel happier, have more abundance or lose weight. Here is how to put the karmic principles of motive, speech, attitude and action into practice:

The first step is **right motive**; let's say you are choosing to be healthier by losing weight.

The second step is **right speech**; to formulate a simple "I am statement" of what you want, such as:

- I am able to release stress as it arises
- I am choosing food wisely and shedding weight

The next step is **right attitude** which requires focus. Focus your mind on the results you want. You must put your attention on the right attitude for getting the results you desire. Get very clear and specific. The more positive and detailed, the better.

Then brand your statement into your subconscious mind which will be the key to your success. The last step of **right action** is this constant, consistent repetition of your statement which will sustain your focus and lead to your follow through and excellent results.

Memorize your "I am" statement and repeat it daily. Run it constantly through your mind. Feel it, breathe it. Write it out 100 times daily, put a post it note on your dashboard and bathroom mirror. If you are serious about getting real change in your life through reprogramming your subconscious mind - do this.

It is possible to change, but it can take some time. Stay in relaxed awareness of what is happening; you are retraining your brain. Be patient and be persistent.

Be Real

This step of right action correlates to the agreement, always do your best. Remember, when we know that we have done the best job possible and not left anything fall to the side, we feel great. The tricky part is honestly recognizing our capacity and determining the extent of our individual responsibility in any given situation. Our best will vary from day to day, moment to moment and is dependant on our health, emotional state, energy level and the unique situations we face. Always doing our best involves being present and conscious enough to discern what the best plan of action is.

Now you know - will you do it?

Get started down your own path of karma at
www.CatherineMazurYoga.com/karma

Chapter Nineteen
Healing Your Body

*"No matter whether you are happy or sad,
in pain or not in pain, with or without a diagnosis,
there is something unchanging in each of us,
and that is fundamentally our awareness."*

- Gary Kraftsow

Back, neck, and knee, hip and shoulder pain can be caused from a single traumatic event, such as an injury from over stressing or straining the muscles. It can also stem from an energy blockage which is felt as pain in the body. In this chapter, we briefly look at some of the most common sites of physical pain and their root causes.

Back Pain

Most back pain is caused by an accumulation of stress to the soft tissues surrounding the spine which leads to pain and suffering. Our posture and repetitive movements during our daily activity cause an imbalance in our muscles. The pain is caused when a disc presses into a bone, ligament, or nerve.

Many of us sit for a good portion of the day placing the spine in an unnatural position of flexion, or rounding of the back. We may not realize the strain we are putting on our spine because we may not feel the pain until the evening or later that day.

If you bent a finger back further than its natural range of motion for a couple of moments, it most likely won't bother you, but if you hold it like that all day you'll end up in pain. Or if you bent a pen forward and backwards, it wouldn't break the first time. It would remain intact until perhaps the 1,012 time and then on the 1,013, it would snap. It isn't one bend that causes the damage, rather the accumulative stress over time. This is what happens with our backs, necks, knees, hips and shoulders.

Fortunately, many back issues are relieved by the regular practice of yoga. The poses create a balanced strength and flexibility all along the spine and contribute to returning the natural curves to the low back and neck. By lengthening the leg muscles and reversing patterns of improper posture, many back issues are alleviated.

Neck Pain

As we sit stand or walk during the day, we tend to let our neck and head tilt forward, out of alignment with our spine. The head weighs about 10-12 pounds, and this forward head position puts strain on the cervical spine. It can also be the cause of pain or tingling in the arms and fingers, or can eventually lead to a herniated disc in the cervical spine.

Regular yoga promotes body awareness which is a large part of maintaining proper alignment of the head and neck. It will strengthen the muscles of the neck and spine which will improve posture, alleviating your aching neck.

Shoulder Pain

The shoulder joint is a complex ball and socket joint which is relatively unstable and subject to muscular injury. During the day repetitive movements like driving, reaching, and working on the computer keyboard cause an imbalance of the muscles working in the shoulder joint. Like the back and neck, we might not notice it right away, but in time we can develop pain in the shoulder due to the uneven strain in the muscles surrounding the shoulder joint and improper alignment when we are using our arms and torso. Alternating between different forms of exercise will help to alleviate a shoulder condition by bringing balance and symmetry to the muscular structure which protects the joint.

Yoga strengthens the surrounding muscle of the shoulder joint and more importantly, it increases your range of motion, which will help to prevent frozen shoulder and similar conditions.

Hip Pain

Like the shoulder, the hip is also a ball and socket joint. The most common cause of hip pain is arthritis, particularly osteoarthritis. These conditions develop over time due to the wear and tear on the joint.

Another common cause of hip pain is tendinitis and bursitis. Many tendons around the hip connect the muscles to the joint. These tendons can easily become inflamed if you overuse them or participate in strenuous activities like running, tennis, or soccer. Excess weight can also put pressure on the hip joint, so shedding those extra pounds can provide relief and help you avoid further problems.

Many of the yoga postures target the hips and legs. As flexibility increases, the joints are freed to operate without restriction and hips can be rehabilitated. When hip issues are related to an inflamed tendon or cartilage wear and tear, the increased blood flow to the joint can aid in healing.

Knee Pain

The knee is the largest hinge joint in the body. As with the other joints, muscle strains, tendinitis, arthritis, and everyday wear and tear can contribute to knee pain. Excess weight puts undue stress on this joint. Symptoms of these are pain, limited range of motion, swelling of the joint, tenderness, and weakness. Often problems with the feet or ankles will contribute to the misalignment of the knee joint, causing irregular wear on the cartilage and stress on the ligaments in this complex joint.

Yoga will help to rehabilitate the knee by teaching you correct alignment of the knee joint. As you increase flexibility in the hips, quadriceps and related muscles, you will relieve imbalanced pressure on the knees that comes from tight hips and upper legs.

Osteoarthritis

This is a common condition of inflamed tissue which causes pain in the joints. All of our joints are lined with soft tissue, and when this tissue becomes inflamed it's painful. To offset this condition, we need some level of exercise and stretching, an anti inflammatory diet, and attention to the proper alignment of our spine and limbs.

Crisis or Maintenance

When you experience severe or moderate pain flare up, you must first determine whether it is a muscular problem or a disc problem. Muscular pain will eventually subside whereas a disc problem can be chronic and might need physical therapy.

Either way, during an acute flare up you should avoid vigorous stretching, flexion, and flexion rotation. In addition to your normal daily activity, these movements might heighten your pain rather than relieve it.

When the flare up subsides, resume a maintenance program of regular yoga. Usually about 3 to 4 weeks after the trauma or acute pain is a great time to return to yoga.

Finding The Right Fit

Because there are a variety of yoga styles ranging from gentle to vigorous, it's important to look for an appropriate class. A vigorous style, like bikram, ashtanga,or vinyasa, probably isn't a good choice for chronic sufferers who are in constant pain. A good rule of thumb, the gentler the better. Look for a class geared towards people wanting to rehabilitate. Or a class that emphasizes rest and restoration. As your condition improves, you can reevaluate your yoga practice and choose a style and class that continues to challenge and support you while it meets your needs.

It is important to learn how to modify the poses and use yoga props for any poses that feel beyond your comfort level. Using yoga props, like blocks bolsters and straps, help to bring the poses to you when tight or weak muscles cannot fully bring you to the pose. Think of these props as arm extensions.

It Can Happen To Anyone

In the United States, back pain is one of the most common complaints. The Mayo Clinic states that most people will experience low back pain at sometime in their life. Low back pain is experienced by sedentary people as well as highly trained athletes. If you have a back problem, it's best to get an okay from your doctor before trying any form of exercise.

Back pain is also often the result of a biomechanical imbalance in spinal structures, so you will want to talk to your doctor who can advise you of any movements to avoid, the most productive levels of challenge, and the effects of any interaction between exercise and your medications.

Once you've had a conversation with your doctor, look for an appropriate level yoga class and tell your yoga teacher about your restrictions and your doctor's advice. A good yoga teacher will be able to respond to your physical limitations with the use of props and modifications so that your experience with yoga is safe and beneficial.

There are certain poses that are appropriate and beneficial for just about everybody, despite physical limitations or injuries. These basic, gentle poses move the spine in all six directions, bringing healing to the body.

Go to **www.CatherineMazurYoga.com/sixdirectionyoga** for a video to lead you through this gentle healing flow appropriate for everyone so that you can start feeling better today.

Chapter Twenty

Healing Your Back with Yoga

"The best way out is through."
- Robert Frost

Jenna's Story

In November, my boyfriend (now husband) suggested we give yoga a try. We had both suffered from back pain for awhile. After exploring various workout routines for months, we weren't really falling in love with any of them.

I honestly thought yoga would just be another thing we tested out only to quickly forget about it...boy, was I mistaken! It's been almost three years, and I am still practicing 3-4 times a week. I absolutely love it!

My high anxiety is in check. I no longer have any neck or back pain. Plus, my body is the leanest it has ever been and I actually have some muscle now! Yoga has proven to be more than a workout routine. It is a lifestyle. My lifestyle.

Why It Works

Doing yoga cultivates a balance between flexibility and strength which is often the real culprit in back pain. Most people are tight in areas affecting their spine, namely the hips and shoulders, which can pull the spine out of alignment. Yoga releases muscular tension, which in turn, can definitely improve back pain. The magic of yoga is that it combines stretching and flexibility while it develops muscular strength that supports skeletal alignment.

Muscle development is essential to protecting the bones and joints. As you do the physical poses of yoga, all of the major and minor muscle groups are enlisted. This whole body muscular engagement is another hallmark of yoga. From the large group of four muscles in the front upper leg known as the quadriceps, to the tiny muscles in the hands and feet, everything is called upon in your yoga practice.

A well rounded yoga session will include the stretching and strengthening of opposing muscle groups such as quadriceps and hamstrings, triceps and biceps, tops of the feet and the arches. In strengthening the opposing muscle groups, skeletal integrity is maintained and the joints are stabilized. The spine is supported in its proper symmetry, making it stronger and pain free.

It is this whole body system that results in a healthier back through developing balance, strength, and flexibility as well as body awareness and alignment.

Back pain sufferers need to be especially aware of proper alignment which means the proper location of your body parts in relationship to one another. Proper alignment of your feet, knees, hips and spine will make all the difference as to whether you get deep relief or end up making your condition worse.

By its very nature, yoga is well-suited to address back problems arising from postural alignment conditions such as kyphosis, scoliosis, lordosis, stenosis (narrowing of tissues) and problems with the in vertebral disks. These conditions require modifications and definitely a gentle, prudent approach. However, even a beginner can derive great benefits and get relief.

Emergency Care

For acute pain, the key is to relax your back and to encourage and promote the natural S shaped curve of your spine. If you have a slipped disc in the lower back or sciatica flare up, please avoid all deep forward bends as these can make your condition worse.

Here are some positions guaranteed to make you feel better and relax your back.

- Lie on your back, bending your knees. Place a pillow or yoga blanket under them to support them as you relax your hips and back. This bent knee position releases tension in the low back. If you need more support, place a small rolled up towel under your back.

- Lie on your side and place a pillow or yoga blanket between your knees. Maintain the alignment of your spine by bending your knees to ensure that your ear, shoulder, hip, and ankle are all aligned. Support your head with your hands or a small pillow to keep it in line with your spine.

- As you're resting, be sure to change positions. Avoid maintaining one position for too long which will result in tightening up the spine and joints.

Two things to avoid while you are experiencing acute back pain are abdominal crunches or hamstring stretches. They both flatten the back and put extra pressure on the disks.

Six Soothing Poses For Your Back

- **Prone Prostration** - Lie on your stomach for five to ten minutes. This releases the back and allows the spinal discs to slide back into correct alignment, reversing the overflexion which is a common cause of back pain. It is important to repeat a few times a day.

- **Seal Pose** - Lying on your stomach, bring your hands about 8-10 inches in front of your shoulders and slightly wider than your shoulders. Press into your hands and lift your upper torso while trying to keep your abdominal muscles and glutes soft. Hold your head directly over your shoulders and straighten your arms, looking up. This pose will decrease back pain by sliding everything back into place. First do this pose by flowing up and down five to six times with your breath. After your spine is accustomed to this motion and stretch, stay up for a couple of breaths.

- **Half Locust** - Here we begin to challenge the spine. Staying on your stomach, extend your opposite arm and leg. Lift and hold for a count of five then lower, switching sides. The goal is to hold for thirty seconds. The key is to focus on straightening the knee to keep the work in the back not the hamstrings.

- **Spinal Extension** - Come onto your hands and knees with your hands under your shoulders and knees under hips like a table. Maintaining a neutral position of your spine, extend opposite arm and leg. Keep the spine in a level position as if there was a glass of water on your back. This pose will work your core muscles, shoulders and glutes. Again, the focus is on straightening the leg completely with no bend in the knee to ensure the engaging of the hip and back muscles rather than the hamstrings.

- **Plank** - This is an excellent pose for strengthening your core. It maintains a neutral position of your spine and strengthens all aspects of your midsection, back, sides and front, making it one of the most effective core exercises you can do. To increase the intensity, lift one foot off the ground, keeping the leg straight and hold for the count of five then switch to lift the other leg.

- **Standing Cobra** - With your feet hip width apart, bring your hands onto your lower back, fingers pointing down. Keeping your legs very straight, begin to bend back as far as you can while keeping the low back neutral. It will feel as if you are lifting up from your heart rather than dumping pressure into your low back. Hold for a breath and repeat this five to six times. This is an excellent exercise to rehabilitate your back.

Maintaining A Healthy Back

Here are seven poses I recommend to maintain a healthy back and relieve achy muscles. These seven poses create a twenty minute yoga flow which you can do daily to keep yourself and your back healthy and pain-free.

- **Supine Hamstring Stretch** - Begin by lying on your back with a strap or towel nearby. Draw one knee up and place the strap or towel under the arch of your foot. Holding onto the strap, with the corresponding hand, lie back and begin to straighten the leg. As you do this, allow the strap to slide through your hand, remaining taut. Try to keep the opposite leg and hip connected down towards the floor. Only go to the point where you feel the first initial stretch in your hamstrings, the muscles in the back of your thigh. Flex your right foot by pressing through the heel and curling your toes down towards your face. Contract and squeeze the quadricep muscles in the front of the thigh. Stay here for 5 to 10 deep breaths. Repeat on the other leg.

Benefits: This pose increases the flexibility of your hamstrings and calves. It can help to prevent varicose veins, relieve low back pain, and calm the nervous system.

- **Double Knee Reclining Twist** - Begin by lying on your back with your knees bent and your feet flat on the floor. Hug your knees to your chest, bringing them up one at a time to protect your back. Roll to one side, knees curled in and up. Begin to extend your top arm in the opposite which will initiate a twist in your torso. Hold for five to ten breaths, relaxing your spine and looking in the direction of your top arm. Roll onto your back and lower your feet to the floor one at a time, leaving the knees bent. Repeat on the second side.

Benefits: This deep twist will release your spine and relieve low back discomfort. It stimulates the internal organs and flushes toxins from the system.

- **Hip Opener** - Begin by lying on your back with your knees bent. Cross your right ankle over the left knee making sure that the anklebone clears the thigh and flex your foot. Maintaining alignment, pull your right knee in toward your chest, thread your left arm through the triangle between your legs and clasp your hands around the back of your right leg. Avoid rounding the upper back and use a strap around your thigh if you need one. The goal is to avoid creating tension in the neck and shoulders as you open the hips. As you draw your right leg in toward you, simultaneously press your left knee away from you

Benefits: This pose is an extremely effective hip opener that will increase the external rotation of the femur bone in the hip socket. It also lengthens the psoas muscle that is one of the culprits of back pain. In our chair-bound society, the psoas becomes shortened and tight, pulling on the low back.

- **Cat Cow** - Begin with your hands and knees on the floor in a tabletop position. Start with a neutral spine and your head aligned with your spine. On your exhale, round your spine up towards the ceiling drawing your navel up towards your spine. Press your hands into the floor and tuck your chin towards your chest letting the back of your shoulders stretch and the back of your neck release. On your inhale, look up and let your belly drop towards the floor, arching tailbone up. Continue flowing back-and-forth between this arched pose, cat, and the cow pose, connecting your breath with each movement; inhaling as you look up and exhaling as you tuck your chin and round your spine.

  Benefits: This pose is a wonderful way to start off any yoga practice. It's really a combination of two poses which help to warm up your spine and relieve back or neck tension after a long day.

- **Child's Pose** - Begin by kneeling on your hands and knees in table pose. Point your toes and separate your knees about hip width apart. As you exhale, slowly lower your hips towards your heels. As your torso folds over your thighs, lengthen the back of your neck, bringing your forehead to rest on the floor or a yoga block. Stretch your arms out in front of you with the palms facing down. Stay here for five to ten slow breaths.

Benefits: Stretches the low back, hips, thighs, knees and feet. Relaxes the spine shoulders and neck. Massages your internal organs, increases blood circulation to the head, which calms the mind, reduces headaches, and relieves stress and tension.

Modifications: Bring your arms back by your hips with the palms up. Place a cushion behind your knees if the stretch across the knees is too deep. Place a rolled up towel under your ankles if the stretch is too deep for the ankle or foot.

- **Sphinx Pose** - Lying on your stomach, prop yourself up on your forearms, aligning your elbows directly under your shoulders. Point your toes and press firmly through the tops of your feet bringing all ten of your toenails towards the floor. Press evenly through your forearms and hands, taking care to distribute the weight evenly from thumbs to pinkies. Draw your pubic bone forward and lengthen your tailbone toward your heels. Roll your shoulders back and down to help draw your lower ribs forward. You will feel sensations in your lower back,
  but breathe through it. You are allowing blood flow to your back.

Benefits: Sphinx pose is a gentle backbend which is invigorating to the nervous system. It counters the rounding of the thoracic spine due to poor posture. The chest and shoulders are stretched and released.

- **Downward Facing Dog** - Begin on your hands and knees. Spread your fingers wide and tuck your toes under. On an exhale, lift your knees off the floor and press your hips up and back to make the shape of an upside down V. Gently begin to straighten your legs, pushing your arms forward and drawing your heels towards the floor, feet hip distance apart. Your hands should remain shoulder distance apart with your wrists aligned with the top edge of your mat. Continue to lift through your pelvis and firm the muscles of your arms, pressing your index fingers and thumbs into the floor. Hold for five to ten breaths and release.

Benefits: This pose energizes the entire body. It deeply stretches your hamstrings, shoulders, calves, feet, hands, and spine while building strength in your arms, shoulders, and legs. It is considered a mild inversion because your head is lower than your heart in this pose, and so it holds all the benefits of an inversion: relief from headaches, insomnia, fatigue, and mild depression. The flow of blood to the brain also calms the nervous system, improves memory and concentration, and relieves stress.

- **Legs Up The Wall** - Begin by sitting with the side of your body against the wall. Turn your body to lie on your back and bring your legs up onto the wall. Shift your weight from side to side and draw your hips close to the wall ensuring that you align your spine and level out your shoulders. Let your arms rest at your side with the palms facing up. Close your eyes and hold for five to ten minutes. To release, slide your legs down the wall and roll to your side. Use your hands to help you press back up into a seated position.

Benefits: This post is excellent for relaxing the muscles of the lower back and drains stagnant fluid from the feet and ankles. It quickly rejuvenates the low back and legs, eases tension and helps to boost circulation

Modifications: Use a bolster or blanket underneath your hips to elevate your low back and hips.

The Proof Is In The Relief

Multiple studies document the benefits of yoga for back pain sufferers. In Britain, a three-year study researched the effects of yoga on chronic back pain sufferers. The yoga participants scored much better than the control group in all areas including pain.

Of all the comments that I've heard over the years from my hundreds of students, the most common benefit is that their back pain has subsided or is completely gone.

Yoga certainly does help back pain, but you must respect the limits placed on you by your pain, which involves listening to your body. This is a skill you will undoubtedly cultivate as a student of this ancient system of healthcare.

Yoga will teach you to respect your body and what feels appropriate for you on any given day, rather than comparing your current ability to what you used to do or with what someone else can do.

A unique aspect that yoga offers is mindfulness techniques and the environment in which to work on deeper levels of healing and pain resolution.

Want a five minute yoga routine for back pain relief? Visit
www.CatherineMazurYoga.com/5minuteyoga

Chapter Twenty One
Joint Pain And Autoimmune Disease

"For a seed to achieve its greatest expression,
it must come completely undone. The shell cracks,
its insides come out and everything changes.
To someone who doesn't understand growth,
it would look like complete destruction."

- Marcel Proust

Darcie's Story

I have had fibromyalgia for about 3 years now. I didn't know it at the time, but it started with headaches and they weren't normal headaches. It felt like a sub-woofer was going off in my head. I got a CAT scan done and the results showed nothing wrong. Then, everything started happening one-by-one. The next thing I experienced was pain in my hamstrings, and then horrible pain in my Achilles that couldn't be explained. All the symptoms came separately and at different times.

They say that fibromyalgia can be triggered by something traumatic like an accident or a surgery. Mine started the day my job was downsized. I got moved from a manager to a receptionist, which wouldn't usually bother me, but I started getting bullied daily by the people I worked for, I guess to remind me of my place. I was diagnosed about a year ago because I kept trying to find out what was wrong.

It's hard to explain what it feels like, but I'll start from the top and go down. When the headaches are around, it can be incapacitating, and I can feel my head pulsing. Waking up can be hard when I'm having a flare up and a kind of mental fog settles over me. It can almost feel like you are drunk but haven't had anything to drink, and not the fun drunk either. I have had times when it scared me because it was so hard to wake up. It's hard to go to sleep and hard to wake up. I used to have a problem with insomnia when the symptoms first started, and would stay up for 3 days at a time.

Most of the actual pain, the worst pain, is in my legs. In the upper legs, it becomes a deep pain/ache that can't be reached. It's a constant moving around trying to get comfortable, hoping that a different position will help. If I stay in one position too long, it's like things get stuck and my muscles can get really mad. Most of the pains in my legs are described as tender spots, I call them sore. I typically have a racquetball with me that I will do a trigger point pressure release. It seems to help them relax. The Achilles pain was the worst and the onset was very scary because my dad tore his tendon and that's what I didn't want. I noticed it one day when I was walking/exercising. I sat down and felt around and pushing on the tendon was like a level 12 on a 1-10 scale. It felt like the worst muscle soreness you'd ever had, but it was worse because the tendon is used so much in walking/standing/moving, etc.

I started physical therapy and they gave me all these stretches, including a really good one for the lower part of the calf, which still feels great. But the physical therapy and the two stretches they had me doing didn't do anything to help at all. Sometimes the fibro seemed to attack my joints and everything got itchy. It also seemed to affect my IT band.

The only solution the doctors offered was to give me medicine that changed my brain! That scared me more than anything, and I didn't want to take medicine the rest of my life. I wanted to find a way to hold it back. So, I developed my own physical therapy.

To help with the mental stress and aspects of my condition, I decided to enroll for two acting classes, and a physical improv. The acting helped with the headaches. Something about it made my headaches lessen, but the physical symptoms of fibromyalgia remained. I also started swimming two days a week in an effort to rehabilitate my legs.

I had started doing yoga back in about 2000. I had trained as a dancer, was a cheerleader and was always stretching so I think it kind of naturally started. The small town I'm from didn't have yoga studios, so I started with home dvd's. Most of my practice was at home, and on the road when I travelled working as a flight attendant. I can't remember what city I was in when I went to my first yoga class at a gym.

Now, I work at a youth and teen center on a military base. When I started, the manager asked me about the things I enjoy. Yoga was one of my answers. She invited me to teach the kids and although I had never taught anyone before, I put together something simple and the kids loved it. The staff did too, because it was a nice break in the afternoon to get a good stretch.

I began to consider deepening my yoga practice as a form of rehab and decided to do a 200 hour teacher training intensive to give me the knowledge to be able to practice at any time, anywhere. It isn't always easy for me to get to classes because of full-time work and school, so I thought this training would allow me to do as much as I could when my schedule is tight.

I couldn't wait to start the training!

I purposely didn't do any yoga for about three months before I started teacher training because I wanted to keep my rehab experiment as pure as I could. I needed to know what worked and what didn't. The symptoms were at their worst two months before starting teacher training.

The first weekend was hard. I don't think I'd ever done two hour long classes before and it hurt a great deal. There was a lot of pain in my hamstrings from the stretching. I was very sore and there were still quite a few symptoms that remained.

On Monday, at work, the headache didn't come and when I realized that, I noticed I didn't have pain in my Achilles. When I actually pressed against them they were at about a level 3, but they weren't throbbing. After the next weekend, the Achilles pain was gone, and though I was sore from yoga, it wasn't the scary sore that had been in my hamstrings. I think the soreness and the intensity going down as I kept practicing was possibly scar tissue being worked out.

By the third or fourth week of the training, the pains from the fibro were gone. Even though I had been having some major pains on my right side, IT band, plantar fasciitis, numbness, etc....it all went away. And even as I sit here now, I just checked my Achilles and there is zero pain. There is no pain in my legs, no deep ache.

I think I opened up some pathways that were blocked. The energy pathways really speak to me, and that was my first personal experience of seeing what happens when they are blocked and then reopened.

I met with someone today who did diagnose me with hypothyroidism, which I've always known. But I'm sure I'm on the right path and I think as long as I continue forward, my weight will catch up to me. Last week, I pushed up into a full backbend, urdhva dhanurasana, and it felt so amazing.

I'm in a transitional phase to follow a career that is healthier and active. I hope that being a teacher can help me do that. I'm happy I challenged myself with the teacher training and experienced first hand the healing power of yoga. I plan to make yoga not just something I practice for myself, but an integral part of my life as I share with others its ability to rehabilitate autoimmune conditions like mine.

Yoga For The Immune System

Ten million Americans are coping with an autoimmune disorder, which is a term encompasses more than 80 conditions including Graves' disease, rheumatoid arthritis, lupus, and multiple sclerosis. An autoimmune disease occurs when the immune system turns on the body, misidentifying normal cells as invaders. The normal cells being attacked could be connective tissues, like in lupus; or the nerves, as with MS; or the joints, as with rheumatoid arthritis.

Yoga can address some of the physical and mental challenges for those dealing with diseases that compromise the immune system. On a physical level, studies show that yoga stimulates the parasympathetic nervous system which has a calming effect, and profoundly affects the immune system.

Specialists agree that yoga can also help ease the psychological challenges of living with a chronic condition. "One of yoga's most important gifts is an inner connection to the reality that you are not your diagnosis," says Gary Kraftsow, founder of the American Viniyoga Institute. "People suffering from autoimmune disorders need to shift their fixation away from the body to something that is deeper and unchanging. No matter whether you are happy or sad, in pain or not in pain, with or without a diagnosis, there is something unchanging in each of us, and that is fundamentally our awareness."

A small study published in the medical journal, *Alternative Therapies*, showed that in a 10 weeks study, women in the yoga group reported better balance, less pain, and also experienced less depression than those in the control group.

Is this because yoga helped them reconnect with their bodies in a meaningful way?

Learning how to relate to the body in a compassionate way can be very healing. Listening to our bodies and taking care of them with love and devotion will open up an energy flow within us. Any form of yoga whether it's restorative poses, vinyasa flow, hot yoga or the practice of meditation and contemplation, can be effective in relieving the symptoms of autoimmune disease.

For information and a link to the teacher training program that changed Darcie's life, visit the link at
www.CatherineMazurYoga.com/teachertraining

Chapter Twenty Two

7 Steps To Better Health

"To take one step is courageous;
to stay on the path day after day
choosing the unknown and facing yet another fear,
that is nothing short of grace."

- Danna Faulds

In this chapter, you will learn simple, effective ways to be proactive about taking care of your mind, body, soul and spirit. They are simple, quick and they will get your day off to a great start.

The following steps are my top recommended proactive daily habits. They can easily be done in the first twenty minutes of your day.

Step #1

THE MOST IMPORTANT 5 MINUTES OF YOUR DAY

Commit 5 minutes every morning to do something meaningful for yourself. We always find time to brush our teeth, and wouldn't feel right if we didn't hop in the shower to take care of our body. If we didn't make the time for these essential personal care habits, we would feel somehow not right, not ready to go out into the world.

There is nothing more important than feeding our spirit and taking care of our mind and soul. So, why do we totally neglect a morning habit to nurture this part of ourselves?

Begin every day with a 5 minute practice to feed your mind, soul and spirit. It could be a devotional reading, a journal entry, meditation, or even listening to an inspiring podcast while you get ready for your day. Choose something that resonates with you that you can commit to. Then watch how it changes the way you enter into your day.

Step #2

DAILY AFFIRMATION

Before your feet hit the floor every morning, create one strong affirmation to declare aloud to yourself such as:

- I am going to have an extraordinary day today!
- I am not influenced by what other people do or don't do!
- I make wonderful decisions!
- I am so grateful that my feet hit the floor today!

Step #3

TONGUE SCRAPE

Head to the bathroom to scrape your tongue; that's right - get a tongue scraper. Dental research has concluded that a tongue scraper is more effective at removing toxins and bacteria from the mouth than a toothbrush.

Step #4

OIL PULLING

Oil pulling, or kavala, is an ancient Ayurvedic dental technique that involves swishing a tablespoon of oil in your mouth for 3 - 20 minutes daily. This action draws out toxins from your body and improves your oral health, which also improves the overall health of your body. The simplest way to do this daily is to keep a pure oil, either sesame or coconut oil, and a spoon in your bathroom cabinet. After you've scraped your tongue, put the oil in your mouth and roll it around while you fix your hair, makeup and dress for the day. Spit the oil out into the trash or toilet (not your sink, where the oil may solidify and block up the drain) and rinse with warm water. Your teeth will be whiter and your gums healthier.

Step #5

CAYENNE LEMON WATER

Pour a large glass of room temperature purified water and squeeze half of a lemon into it. Shake a tiny bit of cayenne pepper in to aid your body in detoxing and rev up your internal heat for the day ahead. While you drink the water, mentally repeat your affirmation. Water is a powerful conduit and will saturate every cell in your body with your mental message for the day. For an extra boost you can include a teaspoon of organic apple cider vinegar for its probiotic qualities.

Step #6

BOUNCE A BIT

20 little quick heel lifts or a minute of jumping on a rebounder will do wonders to jumpstart and detox your body. There are many benefits of rebounding, including better lymph drainage, weight loss, and cellulite reduction. If it's too early for you to bounce, just jiggle a little. You can repeat your affirmation 20 times while you bounce.

Step #7

ACID/ALKALINE DIET

To enjoy optimum health, the body needs balanced quantities of alkaline substances and acids. Our bodies are an alkaline environment, and every system within us from our cellular function to our digestive health is compromised if this environment becomes too acidic.

How do you know if you have an acid problem? A simple pH test using your saliva or urine will be very revealing. The vast majority of us are not within the healthy pH zone in which the body operates optimally, fighting off disease, inflammation and illness. Illness cannot thrive in the optimal alkaline environment. The zone of optimal health is from pH 7.36 to pH 7.42.

There are various factors which cause the body to become too acidic, one of them is stress and another is diet.

An imbalance can result in health problems ranging from minor skin irritations, chronic fatigue, back pain and depression to arthritis, ulcers, and osteoporosis. The good news is you can easily change the acid/alkaline balance in your body.

Diet plays a fundamental role in acid-alkaline balance because some foods are alkalizing and others are acidifying. Most people consume an abundance of highly processed foods that acidify the body and as a result, they are afflicted with many of the above ailments.

How can you lower acidity through diet? Start with the morning lemon water which is highly alkalizing. Then begin to eliminate processed foods from your pantry and fridge. These are usually the items that are packaged in a box, can or bag.

To ensure that your diet is more alkaline and less acid, follow the rule that if you can't plant it, grow it, or harvest it - avoid it. All fruits and vegetables are alkaline, so if you eat as close to nature as possible you will choose wisely. Sugar, dairy, and meat are highly acidic, so limit or eliminate these from your diet.

I subscribe to the 80/20 rule which means most of the time you are choosing foods that support your health, energy, and life force. Remember to allow yourself the pleasure of your favorite treats occasionally - Grandma's pecan pie on Thanksgiving, an ice cream date with your kids, or a Friday night pizza.

There are a host of resources to help you navigate your way to a healthier, more alkaline diet. This one health habit alone can affect your life in a very profound way - turning chronic conditions and worsening ailments into non-issues, simply by changing your diet from acid based to alkaline based.

Take Action!

In this chapter you learned many strategies that are simple and easy to incorporate into your daily routine. They pay off big! For additional ideas and resources, please visit my website, **www.CatherineMazurYoga.com/alkaline** where I give you a reference guide of alkaline and acid producing foods and the most important foods to always buy organically grown.

Chapter Twenty Three

Managing Stress With Yoga

"Stress level: extreme.
It's like she was a jar with the lid screwed on too tight,
and inside the jar were pickles, angry pickles,
and they were fermenting, and about to explode."
- Fiona Wood, *Six Impossible Things*

My Vacation Stressed Me Out

Stress can show up as a byproduct of excitement, as when we are excitedly looking forward to doing something new, like an upcoming trip to Bali.

Bob was a "road warrior" and went wherever his company sent him 100 days out of the year. The corporate travel department arranged all the details and he just got on the plane, was chauffeured to his meetings and checked into prearranged hotels at the end of the day.

Everyone thought he had an exciting and extravagant lifestyle, but as anyone who travels for a living knows, it is no picnic. It was a tough schedule, and he definitely felt the stress of his traveling lifestyle.

When he decided to take two weeks to get away from it all and relax in Bali, he made all the arrangements himself, researched all the options, and hoped he was making the right choices. As the trip got closer, he told me that he didn't know if the knot in his stomach was excitement or fear.

When he returned to yoga class after his trip, he sported a great tan and seemed relaxed and renewed, but confessed he felt he needed a vacation to get over his vacation.

There is good stress and not so good stress. Some stress is beneficial and can be an incentive to accomplish a necessary goal. Our bodies respond in the same way whether we are confronted with a challenge we are looking forward to or one that we dread. The nervous system doesn't differentiate between the excitement of something we are up for or the things we resist.

Anytime there is something new on the horizon, our brains prepare our bodies for the upcoming new action by sending neurotransmitters to our body. Neurotransmitters are brain chemicals that communicate information throughout our brains and bodies.

Your body is hardwired to react to any stress in ways meant to protect you. Historically, these stresses showed up in the form of threats from predators; you know, lions and tigers and bears, oh my! Even though the threat of being chased by a tiger is rare today, your body still reacts in the same way to anything that your brain perceives as potentially dangerous or challenging.

According to an article in the *Dartmouth Undergraduate Journal of Science,*

High levels of stress even over a relatively short period of time and in vastly different contexts tend to produce similar negative results such as prolonged healing times, reduction in ability to cope, and heightened vulnerability to infection.

In a normal environment, the brain uses neurotransmitters to tell our heart to beat, our lungs to breathe and our stomach to secrete digestive enzymes. Alternately, under stress, it will send these chemical messengers to elevate the heart rate, stop digestion and make our skin to sweat profusely. These changes to our metabolism and physiology are helpful when being chased by a tiger, but not so much when you can't find the keys to the car or are stuck in traffic.

The world we live in is rapidly changing, our lives are faster and fuller than a decade ago. There is always a new technology, a faster, better way to learn to do familiar jobs. Even turning on the television can be an adventure in navigating applications and figuring out remote controls.

Chronic stress can deplete the levels of neurotransmitters, causing adverse symptoms when they're out of balance. These symptoms show up as eating disorders and insomnia. According to a report by the American Psychological Association, 86% of Americans are estimated to have sub optimal neurotransmitter levels. This can be attributed to our modern lifestyle. We face multiple demands each day as we shoulder huge workloads, try to make ends meet, take care of our families and figure out that darn remote control. Unless we interrupt the stress cycle, our bodies remain in a heightened state of defense.

Ouch, My Ego Hurts

Even more disturbing is the way stress affects our egos. Yes, our egos take a hit when we're under extreme stress. Our brain becomes foggy from the effects of stress, and we don't think as sharply as we would under normal circumstances. This impaired thinking affects our memory and reasoning - which can really embarrass us!

High stress levels have also been linked to the accumulation of abdominal fat. This isn't good for our cardiovascular health or our egos.

This is definitely something we need to change!

Aside from the array of physical benefits, one of the main benefits of yoga is how it helps us manage stress.

Do A Body Check In

Right now, close your eyes and check in with your body. How is your posture? Are you chewing on your lip or jiggling your foot? Notice where you feel tension. Your shoulders or low back?

This is the first step to self awareness - a simple body check in. Doing yoga postures will heighten your sense of body awareness as you hold the poses and feel the micro changes that occur.

Val says the following:

Practicing yoga quiets my mind. It slows down the chatter and allows me to be still. Whether I'm in a pose for an extra breath and noticing what I am feeling or holding in my body and how I react to that feeling...or sitting quietly in meditation connecting to something so much bigger than me.

Yoga connects my physical, mental, emotional, energetic and spiritual self and has opened my heart to live a more authentic life with a stronger connection to my divine. Yoga moves me through fear and resistance and brings my mind and body to a higher vibration. It's a practice where my truths don't need to be spoken out loud or explained because they just are - if I allow them to BE.

It's a place of physical, mental and spiritual manifestations and when I find myself dropping into old patterns or lower vibrations, I go to my yoga toolbox and refocus on breath, being present and taking brief moments of stillness and lengthening them and from there...I begin again.

Stress And Hormones

Stress also greatly affects our hormones, including the hormone cortisol, which is produced by the adrenal glands. When life is too stressful, your adrenal glands may become overworked or fatigued, creating a hormonal imbalance.

When the brain sends neurotransmitters to the adrenals to prepare for a challenge, they release cortisol. Heightened levels of cortisol have been known to have devastating effects on the body and mind. Chronically elevated levels can lead to suppressed immune function, weight gain, blood sugar imbalances, cardiovascular disease, fertility issues, chronic tiredness, trouble thinking clearly and staying on task.

After a perceived threat has passed, our cortisol levels should return to normal; heart rate and blood pressure return to baseline. However, if our stressors are always present and we constantly feel under attack, our fight or flight reaction stays turned on. This overexposure to cortisol and other stress hormones can affect almost all of our body's defenses so it is extremely important to learn healthy ways to cope with stressors in your life.

Which brings us to yoga.

Because the effects of stress show up in many ways, yoga is the ideal solution for the high stress lifestyle we live in and can greatly relieve symptoms that manifest as back pain, hormonal imbalances, weight gain, and brain fog.

Moving your body in coordination with your breath sends a message to your nervous system to relax, giving you relief. The yoga poses specifically target muscles that tense under pressure, so after a yoga session your body feels calm and your mind feels clear. Learning to tame your worrisome thoughts and learning to practice self awareness are the last nail in the coffin of your chronic stress habit.

Using yoga's three main tools, breath, body, and mind, you will definitely get relief from the effects of stress. These three tools use the nervous system to flip the switch from working against you, to working for you. You can get further in depth help in using the three tools by following the links I've provided at the end of each chapter.

Whether your stress symptoms are physical, like back or neck pain, or they show up as sleeping problems, headaches, inability to concentrate or weight gain, yoga offers a toolbox full of customized ways to help you heal.

In addition to healing your body, it is a very effective system for developing and improving coping skills to reach a more positive outlook on life.

For the top five yoga poses to relieve stress visit my website
www.CatherineMazurYoga.com/topfiveposes

Chapter Twenty Four
Moving In The World

*"She could never go back and
make some of the details pretty.
All she could do was move forward
and make the whole beautiful."*
- Terri St. Cloud, *Bone Sigh Arts*

*S*ynthia had been a meth addict for 12 years. When she reached her 27th birthday, she was terrified that she wouldn't see her 28th.

70 pounds overweight, living in abandoned houses with homeless people, and all her money going to buy drugs, she was a long way from her roots.

A good girl, who loved her family and singing in the choir, she had never been a troublemaker. She could have been a rebel though, because her dad, a recovered alcoholic, had given up his addiction, but had never changed his abusive habits. Growing up, she knew she was loved, but harbored a lot of anger for the abuse she endured.

She had always been a large girl and struggled with her body type, wanting to be thin like all the supermodels paraded on the magazine covers. When a friend told her, "I've got something that will stop you from eating all day long," she didn't give it a second thought. At

17 years old, she did her first line of meth. Her friend didn't tell her all the other things it would do.

When she did her second line, she was hooked. At 18, Synthia moved out, which broke her mom's heart, and moved in with her cousin who was also an addict. She lived a hard life, a bad life, but whenever she thought about quitting, the drug would literally call her by name, like a demon. "Synthia, you know you want me," she would hear it say. She felt its presence, like an evil entity.

Synthia managed to put herself through school to be a hairdresser and built up enough clientele to support her drug habit. She met Danny at 26 and told him she was a "really bad addict," but he loved her and they moved in together and tried to make it work.

After three months, her meth habit got even worse and he left her. A couple of dysfunctional relationships and lost pregnancies followed as she continued her downhill slide. She never did heroin though; she had her boundaries. Deep within, she held onto the hope that somehow, someway she would be able to pull herself out of the hell she had sunk into. But meth is a cruel master and after running her business into the ground and losing all her clients, she barely recognized herself. She looked in the mirror and said, "I hate you - I don't even know you."

This 14 year binge left her exhausted and she prayed to ask God to kill her because she couldn't do it anymore. She prayed to be taken home. Her parents were praying for the same release. Every minute, every hour she prayed for it.

Then grace intervened. She had been seeing Danny off and on. When, at 28, she became pregnant again, she felt an uncanny and immediate release. All of her desires and addictions were gone. Just gone. Her deep faith and belief in family arose from the ashes of her life as the answer to her prayers. She focused on her health in preparation to become the best mother she could be and never looked back.

As she stayed clean, she was able to look at the deep anger she had hidden in her heart. This time, a girlfriend invited her to try yoga and she agreed. On their search for a class, they passed a sign for a place called Peace Love and Yoga. They looked at each other and smiled, pulled in and began their yoga journey at PLAY in Carlsbad, CA.

Synthia continued to go to yoga. As she did, she peeled away the layers of anger and grief. One class, in savasana, the final resting pose, she felt everyone else in the room fade away and it seemed like she was all by herself as she heard, "Just let go, you have everything that you need to know and are everything that you need to be. Just let go!"

It pierced her soul. It was like someone went inside and touched her and said, "You are done. You are done with your anger."

I remember her getting up and leaving class that day to compose herself. She knew it had been a hard journey, but a good journey, and now she was headed in a whole new direction.

You're The Programmer, Write The Program

There is a certain point when everything changes. As we become more self aware, many of us discover ineffective scripts, deeply embedded habits that are totally unworthy of us, totally incongruent with the things we really value in life. We find ourselves, like Synthia, living in ways that are very far from who we really are and what we really want. When Synthia got pregnant, there was a chasmic shift within her and she reconnected to what was of ultimate importance to her. She realigned with her life's course and miraculously reclaimed her life.

One of the most effective ways to rewrite your ineffective scripts is to create a personal mission statement or creed. This is a highly personal statement of an unchanging core within you.

In order to write an effective mission statement for yourself, you must start by taking an honest look at how you have been living. What have you put at the center of your life? Is it your family? Your career? Your faith? Yourself?

Sometimes it's not easy to see where you stand and what most greatly influences your life. Often a person will fluctuate from one center to another, resulting in a roller coaster experience of life.

A meth addict's addiction is the center of their life - but as Synthia discovered, there was something deeper and more powerful beneath that center. It was a principle.

If we create our mission statement based on a principle, a deep, fundamental truth, we discover the personal power that is aligned with the way things really are. Our mission statement will have the power of a self aware, proactive individual who is unrestricted by the attitudes and actions of others or by the circumstances and influences that limit other people.

GOALS

The purpose of having a goal is to grow in the direction of your life's mission statement. From time to time, look back upon your choices for the month or the year.

What's worked? What didn't? Where did you get off track?

Putting this into yogic framework, you could ask yourself what karmic seeds did you sow that grew to be pretty nice looking plants? Which were just chaotic weeds? Looking ahead, what would you do differently?

Be careful about the goals that you set, make sure they align with your big picture and life vision. Setting goals that are outside your mission statement will dilute your happiness and your impact in the world. Choose goals that take you in the direction you want your life to go and that stem from your personal convictions. Examine each goal, big and small to discern if it truly something you want or if it stems from outside influences, rather than internal ones.

Quit doing anything that is sucking the life out of you. As you say "No more" to what's no longer true for you, you can ask, "Now what?" and create what matters to you.

EARTH KARMA

Karma, the path of action, takes into consideration the environment, which consists of the entire community of mankind and includes our planet earth. A conscious yogi will try to be informed and aware of how their choices affect humanity and the planet.

Thoughtful use of the earth's resources is a way to acknowledge our interdependence with one another and the planet we share. It is an act of humility and gratitude to use earth's natural resources in a responsible way. Start with habits that are simple to change - turning off the water while you brush your teeth, recycling, planting a tree. As we each try to leave a smaller energy footprint, it can add up to make a big difference. Don't leave it to others. Take responsibility for one or two small changes in your own life.

Supporting the community of mankind can be a tricky choice. It is not always clear which products and services will be a support and which destroy. Insofar as you can determine, be responsible to avoid products that destroy the environment, exploit workers, or undermine your local economy.

Although it isn't always evident, we need to do our best to see how our buying choices affect others.

Do the research on a product before you invest.

- Does this product support my values?
- Does it adversely affect the environment?
- Does it support my community?

LOVE IS A VERB

The way you take action and move in the world is part of your path of karma. In addition to making responsible buying choices, make it your habit to donate your time, talents or resources to those in need.

Do one small thing. Don't overwhelm yourself - that just backfires and you end up not doing anything at all. Instead, make it something you definitely can and will do. Call Goodwill for a donation pickup, do a beach cleanup with some friends, invite an elderly neighbor for dinner. Plan it, schedule it in, put it on your calendar and DO IT!

To create a meaningful vision statement for your own life visit
www.CatherineMazurYoga.com/missionstatement

PART FOUR

THE HEART

*"Allow yourself to experience
every note the heart can play."*

- Michael Singer

Love!

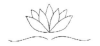

Chapter Twenty Five

The Path Of Devotion

*"The day you were born a ladder was set up
to help you escape from this world."*

- Rumi

*C*hristy's words guided the group as we sat with eyes closed. She was introducing us to the process of connecting to our divine self. *"Your divine self is always sending you support, light and love. All you need to do is to open to it - frequently and consciously."*

"First create the intention to open, then relax into it. There is nothing to do, no efforting here. This connection happens beyond the mind, so whether we feel something or not is not an indication. We only need to set an intention to make the connection and be receptive."

"Let go of thoughts and open to all that is. Let your mind take a state of inner stillness. Ask to be drawn in and then notice what comes up."

Sitting in stillness, I felt all the concerns I had about my life, the trivial and the serious, begin to fall away and I had a sense of entering into a field of universal energy. Swirling, endless possibilities, unfathomable love and support for whatever area of life I chose to explore seemed to open before me. Was this support always available to me without me being aware of it? Am I so busy and distracted with life that I fail to notice the constant support and universal love that holds and guides me?

I decide at that moment to devote myself to opening to this divine force of love and light every day. It makes all the difference.

Bhakti yoga is the path of devotion. This path is wide. It emcompasses all matters of the heart and soul. To nurture ourselves, heart and soul, is one of the highest acts of devotion we can do because we are creators. Each of us creates our own life experience and we all have an influence on others as they create theirs. Never underestimate the power of one life to change the world.

The path of devotion in this section should not be be confused with any religious or spiritual path. Religious or spiritual beliefs are highly personal and do not conflict with Bhakti yoga. Rather, this devotional path is part of and in addition to whatever spiritual tradition you follow. This path is about your devotion to supporting your unique energy, your heart and soul.

Devoted To Being Your Best

If you are depleted and broken, you don't have much to give. Build yourself up to be the best that you can be and in that way you will best serve others and impact the world around you. This focus on meeting your own needs as an act of devotion is the first step to being devoted to any cause or purpose.

In the following section, you will learn how to heal and support yourself through breath, diet, music, media and relationships. We will delve into specific things you can do daily to increase your energy and personal happiness.

As you learn how to nourish yourself, you will become empowered. In the following chapters and the links to the bonus material at the end of each chapter you will learn to maximize the:

- 3 types of energy
- 7 power centers
- 4th agreement
- Power of music

Download a free action plan worksheet to use
as you start down the Bhakti path today at
www.CatherineMazurYoga.com/bhakti

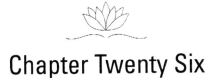

Chapter Twenty Six

Devotion To Your Lifeforce

"The breath is the movement of spirit in the body."
-Andrew Weil, MD

The power of yoga begins in the breath.

There are a variety of breathing techniques that are known to reduce stress, aid in digestion, improve sleep, and cool you down. You can learn to harness the power of your breath to change your emotional, mental, and physical health. Let's look at all three.

Breath And Physical Health

The body, in a living state, breathes involuntarily whether we are awake, sleeping, or actively exercising. Breathing is living. It is a vital function of life.

We can live for weeks without food, days without water, but only a few minutes without breath. Breathing is vital for every cellular function and central to our human life.

Every cell in our bodies need oxygen to function properly. So, it's no surprise that research shows that a regular practice of controlled breathing can decrease the effects of stress on the body and increase overall physical and mental health.

But we don't use all the breathing capacities that our body offers. Instead of using our full lungs' capacity, we breathe quickly and superficially without complete use of the most important muscle for breathing – the diaphragm.

Why is this muscle so important? It is one of the secrets to good health.

The diaphragm separates the chest cavity from the abdomen. With every inhalation, it draws downward into the abdomen and expands the ribcage in all directions. By this movement, air is drawn into all parts of lungs, the abdominal contents are slightly compressed and abdominal pressure increases.

By compressing the abdomen, it massages and stimulates our digestion and increases blood circulation to the abdominal organs. By increasing the pressure inside the abdomen and at the same time lowering the pressure in the chest cavity (as happens with each inhalation), a pressure difference arises between abdomen and chest and that intensifies the blood flow from the abdomen to the heart.

This is pretty important stuff!

By breathing properly and using the diaphragm completely, we inhale greater amounts of air, improve our circulation, strengthen the heart muscle and lungs, and improve and speed up the digestion process. As we speed up the digestive process we balance the levels of fats in the blood which in the long term lowers the incidence of heart attack and stroke.

Additionally, we can also observe a positive influence on the function of the liver, spleen and pancreas. With a better functioning pancreas, the blood sugar level is balanced, lowering the incidence of late-onset diabetes.

Breathing To Heal Cancer

Cancer cells hate oxygen. At least that's what biochemist Otto Warburg discovered. He was awarded the Nobel Prize in medicine for his work demonstrating that all forms of cancer have two basic conditions: high acidity and lack of oxygen. "All normal cells require oxygen, but cancer cells can live without oxygen. Deprive a cell of it's oxygen and it may become cancerous."

Dr. Warburg made it clear the the root cause of cancer is oxygen deficiency and that cancer cells do not breathe oxygen and can't survive in the presence of high levels of oxygen, as found in an alkaline state.

Oxygen heals. In addition to the benefits of increased oxygen in the blood to prevent and heal cancer, there are other beneficial chemicals which are released into our system also, such as endorphins, adrenaline and insulin, which results in elevated emotional states and mental clarity.

Breath And Mental Health

Take a moment now and pause to take three slow, deep, even and quiet breaths. Make the inhales and exhales the same duration, counting as you breathe. Notice how you immediately feel the calming, grounding energy of this short simple exercise.

Because breathing is one of the few bodily functions which can be controlled both consciously and unconsciously, working with breath proves to be life changing. It can connect your conscious mind to your unconscious mind. Breathing is a secret key that unlocks an inner control room to changing your brain!

The unconscious action of breathing is controlled in the brainstem, which automatically regulates the rate and depth of breathing depending on the body's needs at any time. We breathe whether we think about it or not, awake or asleep. It is like our heart which beats 24/7 every day of our life, whether we notice it or not.

The difference between the heart and breath is that we don't have conscious neural pathways to master the control of our heartbeat. However, we do have the ability for conscious breath control. The conscious control of breathing is commonly practiced in meditation and yoga and is called pranayama. It is one of the eight limbs of Patanjali's yoga, as discussed in previous chapters.

Yoga's incorporation of breathing works behind the scenes to affect our brains and to shift deep patterns that we have held for many years. This focus on breathing also brings healing to the body and provides mental well-being. Conscious breathing is the first important step to reclaiming your mind and creating what you want in life, instead of letting the subconscious mind call the shots.

As we focus on breathing, we ignite an awareness that reaches into the subconscious mind. Just by working with conscious breathing we can begin to unhinge deeply held habits and patterns that we want to release. It is through breathwork, or pranayama, that the shift begins to occur.

When our breath becomes a conscious tool, we can free ourselves from our past conditioning and all of the emotional states holding us captive.

Breath And Emotional Health

Our breath not only carries oxygen to the bloodstream to nourish the cells, there is another vital element coming into us to nourish our life. This vital element is prana, or life force, being carried in to nourish our body and soul. In yoga, we refer to breathing as pranayama. <u>Prana</u> is a Sanskrit word that means life force, and <u>ayama</u> means extending or stretching. Thus, pranayama is the extension of breath.

Prana, or universal life force energy, is known in various cultures by different names. It is also known as Qi, mana, shakti, chi, or spirit. It is this life force that we manipulate through yoga. Using our bodies, minds and our breath, we magnify our life force which creates energy and health in our body, mind and soul. Whether we call it emotion, prana, or spirit, our human bodies receive life force with every breath.

Get "In"Spired

The technical term for breathing out is exhalation or expire, which is also the word we use for death or endings. Breathing in is called inhalation or to inspire. Notice the relationship between prana and these definitions of the word "inspiration":

- The act of drawing in; specifically, the drawing of air into the lungs
- A divine influence or action on a person
- The action or power of moving the intellect or emotions
- The act of influencing

Truly, to take a breath is to be inspired!

Yoga incorporates breathing techniques that will relieve stress in your body and help you get through the challenge of any stretch - physically, mentally or emotionally! You can use breath to energize or calm your nervous system, cool or generate internal heat, slow or quicken your heart rate, and to change your mental state. Breathing is truly what distinguishes hatha yoga from other forms of exercise.

Powerful Breathing Exercise

Ever notice how soothing a simple sigh can be at the end of a long day? It is the most natural way to release stress and is a great example of using your breath to change your state.

Here is a simple technique to put your body and mind into a more relaxed and calm state:

- Begin by sitting in a relaxed position
- First breathe slowly, deeply and evenly for three complete breaths
- Next, extend your exhalations, making them twice as long as the inhalations
- Continue for five to ten breaths

Modify the length of your breath to something that works for you. The most important thing is that the exhale is longer than the inhale, not the absolute length of the breath. This breathing technique has a very relaxing effect on the autonomic nervous system.

Practice breathing like this each day for at least 5 minutes. Better yet, pause to practice it throughout your day.

How It Works

Allowing the exhale to last even a few counts longer than your inhale sends a signal along the vagus nerve, which is an important nerve that runs from the brain down the neck through the diaphragm. This signal from the vagus nerve signals the brain to turn up your parasympathetic nervous system and turn down your sympathetic nervous system.

The parasympathetic side of our nervous system is vital in controlling the response to rest, relax, and digest. When the parasympathetic system is dominant, the breathing slows, the heart rate drops, the blood pressure lowers as the blood vessels relax, and the body is put into a state of calm and healing.

Action Step

Remind yourself to breath fully every morning when you awaken and every night as your head rests on the pillow. As you incorporate this breath exercise into your life and use it throughout the day it will produce wonderful health benefits and will help you discipline yourself to become aware of your breathing patterns. You will be able to see a difference in your mood and overall sense of calm!

For a breathing exercise that will give you energy
throughout your day, visit
www.CatherineMazurYoga.com/breathing

Chapter Twenty Seven

Devotion To Your Three Inner Energies

"I want to be thoroughly used up when I die,
for the harder I work the more I live.
I rejoice in life for its own sake.
Life is no "brief candle" for me.
It is a sort of splendid torch which
I have got hold of for the moment,
and I want to make it burn as brightly as possible
before handing it on to future generations."

– George Bernard Shaw

Rob's Story

At 49 years old, Rob went to the doctor for extreme shortness of breath
with physical exertion. When the test results came back they showed all
four major arteries were blocked. Two of them were 100% blocked, one
was 85% and the other 60% blocked.

What the test results couldn't see was that he had suffered in
an unhappy marriage for many years and those who knew him
well believed that after years of feeling unloved his heart energy

was depleted and undernourished. Not feeling acknowledged or appreciated created a negativity which resulted in emotional and physiological effects, his severe blockages being one of them. His lifeforce was literally being cut off as his arteries clogged, mirroring the stagnant flow of energy to his heart.

A few years after his heart procedure, the marriage ended. Rob went on to find the love of his life and has had no regression or heart issues since then.

Bhakti yoga is the path of the soul.

The heart of devotion, the soul, is the unseen energy that makes each of us unique. This energy can be open and flowing or it can be stagnant and blocked. The good news is that energy is always in motion, and we have the power to direct it.

The soul is changeable; it is our nature and personality, existing on an unseen energetic level. There are numerous currents of energy running throughout us; electrical, chemical and emotional. As we begin to see and understand the other unseen but measurable energies in our body, it helps us fathom the unseen energy of the soul which resides in a mysterious dimension and cannot be measured, only experienced.

In exploring the three primary energies of our body, we begin to get a sense of the power and energy of our invisible soul.

Not Our Bodies

We strongly identify with our bodies, referring to them as "my body, my arm, my heart." Stop to think, who is the "my" in mine? This is the Self, or soul, the part that IS you which remains over the years as your body and mind change.

Your body is the soul's earthly residence. The body feels solid, but is just an outer mantle over a spacious energy field which is manifested in this physical dimension. The soul uses the body for expression; though they are separate, they are so intimately connected that we often don't realize how much one affects the other.

Energies That Power Your Body And Soul

While we live in our bodies, we basically utilize three types of energy. Yoga has an affect on all of them. Yoga moves energy through the body and will affect all three of our primary energies; our chemical energy as we burn calories, our electronic energy as we slow heart and brain activity, and our subtle energy which affects our emotions and mood.

Electric Energy

Our nervous system is an invisible highway - an electronic highway.

Nerve pulses are electrical energy signals, a wave of electric activity that passes from one end of the nerve to another. Billions of nerve impulses travel through the human brain and nervous system.

A gigantic network of cells or neurons makes up our nervous system, transmitting information in the form of electrical signals. Electric currents flow through our nerves and every cell in our body. Each cell contains a positive and negative charge.

Polarity exists everywhere in the universe!

Where does this electricity come from? All the elements we take in like oxygen, calcium, and sodium have a specific electric charge, and the way they react to each other creates this human electric energy.

Thought is also invisible electric energy. It is brain energy and somewhat of a mysterious process. Electric sparks fly in the brain, jumping from nerve ending to nerve ending, lighting up our brains like a lightbulb.

In the thought process, our minds regulate the flow of both energy and information. This flow is a movement we can sense and we can learn to direct. It is a dynamic, fluid, moving process that can flow in a direction that is positive and helpful, or become a raging river of negativity and pain. Polarity.

Through the principles of yoga, we can learn to step into the river of our thoughts to change the patterns that are not useful. We can change the course of our life by altering the flow of the river of energy in our mind.

This is one of the powerful tools of yoga. In fact, the very first sutras, or "threads" of Patanjali, relate to the mind and to thought. These first important sutras have nothing to do with mastering advanced yoga poses, and everything to do with mastering the mind.

The Electric Heart

The voltage of the heart is the strongest electromagnetic field in the body, even surpassing the brain. The heart's electromagnetic energy can be detected by instruments from just a few yards away. When the electrical impulses that coordinate heartbeats are not working properly, the heart will beat too fast, too slow or inconsistently.

The heart has a powerful electromagnetic field that generates up to an estimated 60 times the amplitude of the brain. The electromagnetic signal our heart rhythms produce can actually be measured in the brainwaves of people around us.

Not only is the heart the strongest electromagnetic field in the body, it is also the most sensitive organ to subtle energies. The researchers at HeartMath Institute concluded that the heart has its own organized intelligence network enabling it to act independently, learn, remember and produce feelings - all attributes which, until recently, were considered to be solely in the brain's dominion.

Yoga affects the energy of your heart in profound and various ways, from lowering your blood pressure to opening blocked emotional channels.

Chemical Energy

Chemical energy in our bodies is produced from the food that we eat. When we take in food, the large molecules within it are broken down to smaller molecules by our digestive system and those smaller molecules and elements can be used by our cells to do work. Work is measured by calories. When we talk about calories, we are just talking about units of energy. It's a way of describing how much energy our body can get from that particular food.

Here's where we get into trouble though, by consuming more calories, or units of energy, than our body is burning off. What's a body to do? Store those calories in the form of fat cells for a rainy day.

Can't seem to shed that belly fat? In the realm of subtle energy, there is a correlation of the accumulation of abdominal fat to periods of heightened stress or sadness. It is as if the body is protecting the "self" by putting an extra layer of insulation around the core.

Subtle Energy

There are subtle energies within the body that affect everything from our heart to our belly. We feel these energies in various ways, like strong winds blowing through our body which influence our life experience.

We have all felt the energy of emotions, such as anger, joy and despair. Even though we call them subtle energies, our emotions are powerful. They are "energy in motion" and can over overtake us, bypassing all common sense, and drive us to derelict behavior.

We can use these powerful emotions to tune into our soul. Listening to them is our most reliable internal guidance system. They are the closest energy to our soul energy.

Instead of ignoring or suppressing emotional energy, try to become aware of exactly what you are feeling and where you feel it in your body. Turning inward to feel the energy moving through your body can be a powerful ally.

Releasing Strong Emotion

Attention to your emotional energy will help you to process and release the energy in your body. Without this attention, you can easily get stuck on an emotional issue or memory resulting in a lifelong problem. This process is a purely energetic one. It is not a thought process, it is an awareness practice.

When you practice paying attention to the subtle energy in your body you will become free from energy blockages. Staying present with your bodily sensation when you are frustrated, sad or angry will allow the energy to flow through you and be released. By doing this, you will remain free and uninfluenced by the invisible energy of stuck emotions.

Emotions are closely linked to subtle energy of our chakra centers, an intricate system of energy stations and pathways in our body. These pathways and stations have been recognized for centuries in the East, but are slow to be acknowledged by Western medicine. These channels of energy are called nadis or meridians and they are associated with the energy system called the chakras. In the next chapter you will learn about harnessing your chakra energy.

Watch this video for a simple tool to free yourself
from negative emotional energy at
www.CatherineMazurYoga.com/energy

Chapter Twenty Eight

Devotion To Balancing Your Subtle Energies

"Did you know that your brain is
an electronic switching station?
Every cell has both a negative and a positive pole.
You activate brain cells and set up
a vibration in your body. If you activate the negative pole
in any cell, you'll move yourself into a negative vibration.
And when you switch over to the positive pole
you move into a positive vibration."

- Bob Proctor

The word chakra means wheel, or whirling, circular energy. In the body, there are many of these centers whose energy extends out into the organs and limbs, affecting our body, mind and emotions. This chakra energy affects everything about our lives - from our physical health to our behaviors and attitudes.

Traditionally, there are 7 major chakras, aligned vertically up the spine, from tailbone to crown. These centers are powerhouses of energy which govern the entire body. It is helpful to think of the chakras as stations which send out energy along pathways, called nadis or meridians. Just as a train transports goods, the nadis transport energetic information. When these energetic pathways become blocked, there is an unbalance that can be felt as an illness, dis-ease, or emotional and mental discomfort.

In recent years, Western technologies have developed devices that are delicate enough to measure the subtle pulsations of energy along these channels. This proof of subtle energy has changed the way Western medicine thinks. Insurance programs are beginning to recognize and provide coverage for these healing sessions.

Because the chakras are dynamic and changeable energy centers, it is common for them to become unbalanced at some point in our life experience. Our aim is that each of these centers become open and balanced. The practice of yoga can greatly help.

Your 7 Energy Centers

The first chakra is the root chakra, at the base of the spine. It is your foundation and its energetic theme is "I need, I want." It physically governs from the base of your spine to your feet. Root chakra energy relates to all things physical as well as your sense of safety and security, trust, and financial issues. Its color is red.

The second chakra is just above the root, in the lower abdomen. It is your vitality and its energetic theme is "I feel, I sense." All your senses, your lower intestines and reproductive organs are governed by this chakra. It relates to your creative, sensual and emotional self. Its color is orange.

The third chakra is the navel chakra, at the solar plexus, and is your center of personal power. Its theme is "I choose, I will." This energy center relates to your ego, willpower, confidence, intention and self esteem. It is the action center of your energy system and governs digestion and the low back. Its color is yellow

The fourth chakra is the heart chakra, your center of love and connection. Its theme is "I give, I receive." It is your social self and energetically affects your ability to give and receive love, forgiveness, compassion and empathy. Physically, it governs your circulation, heart and breasts. Its color is green or pink.

The fifth chakra is at the throat and is your center of personal communication. Its theme is "I express, I listen." All the ways you express yourself emanate from this energy center. The way you speak, teach, learn, dress, make love and dance are influenced by it. Your neck, throat, jaw, teeth and ears are governed by the fifth chakra. Its color is sky blue.

The sixth chakra is at the brow, often called the third eye. It is your vision and its theme is "I imagine, I see." It affects the upper portion of your head to the tip of your nose, including your brain, nervous system and eyes. Energetically it governs your ability to analyze, dream, reason, discern and perceive. Its color is deep indigo blue.

The seventh chakra is the crown chakra, at the top of your head. It is your connection to all things spiritual and to your highest consciousness. Its theme is "I know, I am." Universal awareness and absolute faith originate from this energy center. It relates to the master gland - the pineal. Its color is violet or white.

For detailed information on the chakras and how to use yoga to balance them, click on the link at the end of this chapter.

The Energy Of Yoga

The real power of yoga lies in using awareness to move and release energy. All forms of yoga will act upon the subtle as well as the major energy systems of your body including your heart, brain, emotions, and chakras. There are many ways you can use energy in yoga, depending on what your focus is and what type of yoga you choose to practice. Within the four main paths of yoga, there are many schools and types.

There are very athletic, physical types of yoga, like ashtanga or power yoga. Other yoga classes will be very restful and restorative. And there are others, like kundalini yoga, that focus on building internal prana, or energy. You can find Rock and Roll yoga, acro-yoga, and even stand up paddle board yoga.

It is important to find and focus on the type, or aspect of, yoga that speaks to you. All of them will shift your energy and give you benefits. When you find the type of yoga that you love and dive into it wholeheartedly, you will begin to shift energy on many different levels and ultimately heal your body, mind, soul and spirit.

Samskaras

Yoga defines blocked energy as samskara. As we've been discussing, when an event is stored in the subconscious mind because we haven't processed it, it leaves a dormant impression. Samskara is the yogic concept that these imprints left on the subconscious mind will color all of our life, our nature, states of mind and our habits.

These unfinished energy patterns or impressions from our past will run our life despite our best intentions. This explains why we get stuck in cycles that we can't seem to break. Past energy stored in your energetic heart center needs to be released in order for you to get free from the cycle.

The practice of yoga will help you to release samskaras as you move through the yoga poses which release energy and open the channels of the body; the nadis and chakras. It isn't just the physical poses that move energy. The practice of self inquiry, meditation and self awareness, all parts of the system of yoga, will help you release negative samskaras and develop positive ones.

Although yoga has changed over the years, with new types and forms emerging every year, it remains a way of using your body and your mind as a portal to heal. Yoga will bring you to know yourself as you truly are which is healing and transforming. We do this by working with energy.

If you are wondering about your own energy centers and how to balance them so you can think clearly, act confidently and feel content, you will be interested in my complete chakra series at **www.CatherineMazurYoga.com/chakras**

Chapter Twenty Nine
Devotion To Your Diet

*"It's bizarre that the produce manager
is more important to my children's health
than the pediatrician."*

- Meryl Streep

Mark's Story

My story is unique because of the experience I had, and its life changing power, just by drastically changing my diet, going from processed food to no processed food, and supplementing with herbs. Well, there's really more to it than that.

I was suffering from headaches and had tried just about everything to get some relief. My father lived in Sedona and went to a health practitioner with a chiropractic background and a specialty in Chinese medicine. Jim Reese was his name and he had helped my step mother tremendously with her health issues.

Jim's wife had an autoimmune disorder that the doctors couldn't diagnose or treat successfully. Through study and strict application of his methods for diet and detoxing, Jim had guided his wife back to health.

He was well known in the community as a healer and an author, so my dad suggested I come out to Sedona and consult with him.

I had no intention of changing my diet; I could care less.

At our initial meeting, I did a whole questionnaire with all the details about my headaches. I'm writing and writing - a whole two page expose on my headaches. I handed it off to him and he just said, "We are going to take you down a path for detox. That's where we're going to start because your body is out of balance."

He gave me a couple books to read which were an important part of the process. He said, "You have to understand why you are doing what you're doing otherwise it's not going to stick."

I began to follow his detox program which was basically not eating anything that I was eating. For six months, all I could eat were vegetables, three proteins - alaskan salmon, free range turkey, and organic eggs, three grains - amaranth, quinoa and millet, the only fats were organic butter, olive, flax or coconut oil. No fruit, no dairy, no breads or pastas, no oils, no other animal protein. I was going to have to get creative. This was a complete shift in how I nourished my body. It was huge.

I began to feel different sometime in the second week. I started to feel clear and light. I had more energy than I had ever felt. Another great benefit was that I got back to my high school weight. My systems worked like clockwork, my headaches went from a three to a one in intensity, and my sense of well being was... well, I had never had a sense of well being before!

I went through a period of time when I felt like I was never going to die. I can't explain it - I know it sounds goofy, but I almost felt immortal - I don't know what it was. I remember at the peak of how great I was feeling, I parked at my office, and walked in on a really warm spring day, feeling like, gosh - this is a whole other existence for me. I just couldn't believe it!

After a couple months, Jim added some herbs and tinctures to rebalance my system.

He told me that I would have an emotional reaction to what he was giving me. It was almost medicinal, it was so healing. During this time, I had two episodes where it was pretty much like I was outside of myself.

One was a confrontation I had with my father, which I had never had the courage to do before. For years, I had been carrying around resentment and anger toward him and had wanted to speak my truth with him, but couldn't ever bring myself to the point of doing it. During the detox program, something happened in me to empower me and I reached this point of conviction and then just did it. I said everything that had been weighing so heavily on my heart for so many years. It turned out to be incredibly healing for both of us and a turning point in our relationship.

And then, the other episode was an out of character extreme action to help my son when all of his college classes for the semester were dropped out of the system. As I set out to correct the clerical mistake and kept hitting dead ends, it seemed hopeless. I never gave up though. I eventually went all the way up the university's chain of command, all the way up to the dean - at home! I would have never done that before - it's not in me to do that kind of stuff, and I just did it.

This nutritional detox and change in my eating habits somehow got me outside of myself. Outside of the small, afraid shell that was built around me.

The other amazing thing was when I went in for my blood work, my numbers were off the charts from where I was before with good cholesterol and bad cholesterol. I was consuming butter like crazy at that time, it felt like by the pound, buttering everything because it was the only thing I could eat that seemed like a treat. Remember, that for six months all I could eat were vegetables; no fruit, no dairy, a little else. Of course, I did cheat a little when I went out to dinner with the family; I would have bread and butter.

After six months, the cleanse and detox was complete and Jim said I could slowly add foods back into my diet. I remember I went into the garage and got the big tin of Danish shortbread cookies that we had received as a Christmas gift from a client. I was so excited. I opened up that canister of cookies and as soon as I got it up to my mouth, I freaked. I put it in my mouth, took a bite and I couldn't spit it out fast enough. It was like pouring a cup of sugar in my mouth. My body totally rejected it. That was an eye opening experience. I thought, wow, you really can get hooked, addicted to sugar. It was amazingly powerful to experience.

During the detox, I could go to the grocery store and walk down the aisle and know I was in the chip aisle just by the smell of rancid oil. Everything was heightened. It was amazing.

When I tell people my story, they say, "Well then, why would you ever quit? Why did you ever stop?" I laugh and tell them, "You try it and then you tell me."

If my life depended on it, it would be a different story, but my life didn't depend on it. I initially just wanted to get rid of my headaches. I had no intention of changing my diet; like I said, I could care less.

Of course, the other amazing thing I learned from it all is that we think the symptom is what we should treat. But it's not about treating the symptoms, it is getting to the root. Reese could care less about my headaches. We didn't have one single discussion about my headaches, not one. Not one time was the word headache brought up. After that long two page questionnaire; in the end, it didn't matter at all.

And now it's been, gosh, almost twenty years, and although I have certainly reverted and regressed during different periods, there are some things that I've really held the line on and I don't doubt it's made the difference. I can certainly tell the difference when I eat awfully. Everything falls apart again. My system gets all screwed up, my neck goes out.

Then I get back on track, semi-fasting, doing a lot of juicing and limiting my consumption, eating raw as much as possible. Then feel myself coming back. It's there, the body knows.

Enlightened Forks And Knifes

The choices you make about what you eat will impact more than just your body weight. In fact, your food choices have just as much to do with your soul as your body.

Why do people choose to be vegan or vegetarian? What about a raw food diet or eating for your blood type? Often it starts for health reasons, like Mark's headache problem, and eventually turns out to be a soul's awakening.

Sometimes our diet choices stem from a philosophical belief like supporting the environment or taking a stand for animal rights. These too are soul issues, heart choices. We vote with our forks.

Becoming gluten free is trendy right now, and for many it is a necessity. The real issue is not always because an individual doesn't tolerate the gluten, but rather that the wheat strains have been so heavily modified, sprayed, and tampered with that our bodies don't recognize them as food anymore. Because they aren't.

Some people's guts are able to withstand the altered foods we are offered in fast food places and mainstream markets, but eventually the body breaks down, with a strange new allergy, a skin condition, or chronic headaches. What are you voting for?

Becoming enlightened about how you nourish yourself is a very practical matter. As we become aware of the impact our choices have on not only our bodies, but also on our soul and our environment, we are faced with the "knowing vs doing" issue.

Will we continue to choose to "feed" ourselves with choices that don't nourish us?

To become your best self, energetic, alive, courageous and focused, I recommend a number of "musts" and "must nots." Below are a few of them.

MUST

READ LABELS

80% LIVE FOODS

PURIFIED WATER

ORGANIC FRUITS/VEGGIES

MUST NOT

GMOs

HYDROGENATED OILS

BHT PRESERVATIVE

MSG

Pick up your free extensive list of must and must nots at
www.CatherineMazurYoga.com/thegoodthebadtheugly

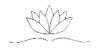

Chapter Thirty

Devotion To Your Dosha

*".…the actual task is to integrate
the two threads of one's life…
the within and the without."*

- Pierre Teilhard de Chardin

Ayurveda is yoga's sister science, a 5,000 year old system of natural healing. It is a holistic system of proactive health care, providing guidelines for daily and seasonal routines, diets and behavior. Ayurveda is the balance and dynamic integration between our environment, mind, body, and spirit.

Mind, body, soul and spirit are found in the environment as fire, earth, water and air. Remember how these relate to the four essential elements which comprise our DNA - carbon, hydrogen, oxygen and nitrogen? The corresponding four paths of yoga mirror mind, body, soul and spirit as the paths of knowledge, action, devotion and meditation.

Ayurveda science looks at three of the four energy types found in nature; the three primary forces of wind, fire, and earth. These three primary forces are called doshas, and they are Vata (wind), Pitta (fire), and Kapha (water).

Each of us has a dominant dosha type and our type will determine which types of activities and health habits will best support our body and our energy. This is a very ancient and intricate science that could be studied for one's entire lifetime. A basic knowledge of your own dosha type can help you maintain or regain your health.

Because our doshas can become out of balance, causing discomfort in our bodies and lives, balancing our primary dosha is an important factor for optimal health. It aids us in making proper choices in our lifestyle and our activities. Knowing your dosha type can guide you to properly nourish yourself. This requires not only monitoring your diet, but also your activities and environment.

Look at the brief description below for each of the three doshas, and see if you can determine what your primary type is.

Three Dosha Types

- Vata, or wind energy, is changeable, light and lively. When Vata energy is balanced there is much creativity and energy, but if it's unbalanced a person can have difficulty focusing and tends to have anxiety.

- Pitta energy is the element of fire and is warm, disciplined, and strong. If it's out of balance, this warmth can become irritable and discipline can turn to compulsion.

- Kapha energy is water. This is an easy-going fluid energy. When kapha is out of balance, a person may be congested and experience sluggishness or weight gain.

This is a vast subject that you might want to explore with an educated ayurvedic practitioner. They can help with a deeper application of this ancient science. Meanwhile, it is helpful to know your particular dosha type and to learn what foods to eat to keep yourself balanced, healthy and happy.

Wondering what dosha type you are? Would you like to know how to support your unique energy type so you feel your best? Go to **www.CatherineMazurYoga.com/dosha** for more info

Chapter Thirty One
Devotion To Your Soul

*"I have found that most people are about as happy
as they make up their minds to be."*
- Abraham Lincoln

*I*n a nursing home for patients with dementia and Alzheimer's, one
resident lies in her bed without speaking and without movement.
*Day after day she barely responds, lying with her eyes closed and her
hands curled into fists. Unresponsive to her family members, the care of
the nurses, or any other external stimuli, she is completely withdrawn,
checked out of the world. She's been there for two years without change,
still alive physically but asleep inside, no longer able to enjoy life.*

*One day, a man enters her room with an iPod and places a headset
on her head. He presses PLAY. Her body begins to soften, a hint of a
smile appears. She starts to shake her head and tap her feet. The nurses
stand there, amazed! Nothing has been able to get through to her until
now. What happened?*

*Music, her music. The songs she danced to as a teenager, when she
was full of life. The sweet songs of love that touched her heart as she
rocked her babies to sleep. Music that was the backdrop of her life seeped*

into the recesses of her mind and woke her up. It ignited something deep inside her, still alive. Music was able to reach where nothing else could.

Alive Inside

What we listen to enters our subconscious mind and ultimately shapes our soul. This is why it is so important to guard your words carefully. They are powerful and once spoken, they can't be taken back. But words aren't the only outside influence that we are strongly affected by.

Take for example, music. The power of music is profound. Have you ever heard a song and it transported you from where you were to another time and place that immediately brought you to tears? Of course you have, music has that power. The switch of a radio station can switch your entire mood, right? From "Amazing Grace" to "Celebrate Good Times," your physiology is influenced by the music you hear.

Music has the ability to activate more parts of the brain than any other stimulus. It strongly links your outer experience to your inner world with the power to uplift you or bring you to tears. The area of the brain that responds to and recalls music is one of the last areas of the brain to succumb to Alzheimer's and other forms of dementia. This is because music connects people to whom they have been and who they are.

In the movie, *Alive Inside*, we follow Dan Cohen on his quest to improve the lives of nursing home patients, especially those suffering from Alzheimer's and other forms of dementia. Cohen's approach is based on findings of neurological scientists that we are hard-wired at birth to "feel the beat."

It all began as we listened to the beat of our own heart in the womb.

Cohen identifies the music most popular in the person's youth; personalizes this music into an iPod playlist tailored to each patient's interests; then puts earphones on these patients and starts their iPods. What happens is remarkable. People who are unresponsive suddenly become alive inside as the music awakens the memories of their lives.

This music phenomena is a tool we can use. We can harness the power of music to access regions in our brains and rewire them. The practice of yoga often includes chanting and singing to shift our state, lift our heart, and nourish our soul.

The Power Of Chanting

From the beginning of mankind, music and chanting have been embedded into human culture. Chanting creates a state of restful alertness. Like an incantation, repeated over and over, it changes your brain. Powerful words spoken with conviction and certainty will engage your physiology in a fashion that unspoken words rolling around in your mind can not. When you speak with certainty and intensity it conditions you and imbeds ideas and nurturing thoughts in your head.

Have you ever had a song stuck in your head and can't get it out? An earworm, some call it. If you have, you know the power of a chant. It gives you a rhythm that impacts you on a deep primordial level.

Chanting is a way to get the right idea into your head. The chanting at the beginning of some yoga classes connects us with a deep part of our humanity. Whether we understand the words or not doesn't matter here. Instead, it's the intensity and vibration that will create a shift. This chanting gets us breathing deeply, rhythmically, and in sync with the others in the room to prepare us for a shift in our body, mind and soul. It is a way to nourish our soul.

What Are You Feeding Your Soul?

A large part of what we nourish ourselves with isn't food.

There is another kind of nourishment which comes in through your eyes and ears. You feed yourself on this for hours every day. Not just the music you listen to, but it is EVERYTHING you're exposed to. All the visual and auditory stimuli you choose during the day enters your brain and has a subtle, or profound, effect on you.

Some things we don't have a choice about. Elevator music. Traffic signals. Sight and sound are the backdrop of our life. All exposure to music, videos, social media posts, games, books, articles, television, radio, conversations, friends - everything that we take in with our eyes and ears goes in and shapes our subconscious. When we become sensitive and aware of the way this external stimuli affects us on a deep subconscious level, we are faced with a choice.

Yes, your mama was right - you are what you eat; whether you are consuming food, Facebook posts or Youtube videos. Do not underestimate the power of those "harmless" lyrics or violent images in the late night movies you are watching. This exposure will have a profound effect on you.

You wouldn't allow a child to watch a disturbing show because you know that it could cause nightmares and fears. Even though your reasoning mind knows the images are only actors and staged sets, your subconscious doesn't differentiate between an image on a tv screen or in real life.

Just food for thought. Actually, the larger consequence of most of the screen time we spend in a day is not a mere nightmare or fear. Its larger consequence is the opportunity lost.

This opportunity is the opportunity of time. When you use some of your down time to feed your heart and soul with fascinating information and uplifting images, music that lightens your mood and podcasts that cause you to challenge your status quo, you are making an investment in your own happiness and freedom.

It's been said that the only difference between who you are today and who you will be five years from now are the books you read and the people you associate with. Think about it.

If you are happy with all the results you are getting in your life, if you feel completely empowered and free, then keep doing the same things. However, if you want your life to be different from the way it is today, if you desire any significant change at all, then you need to bring new ideas and experiences into your consciousness. If you want something you've never had before, you must do things that you've never done before.

Stimulate your mind, body, soul and spirit with inspiring, uplifting visuals. Have engaging conversations with people who challenge you. Listen to fascinating podcasts, such as Tim Ferriss, whose interviews with amazing people will blow your mind; thought leaders like Tony Robbins, New York Times best selling authors, world class chess champions, athletes, geniuses and millionaires.

Hang out with these people for an hour and come away charged and inspired.

Your Tribe

"You'll know a man by the company he keeps."

The people in your life - friends, family, teachers, and co-workers - have an influence your thoughts and behavior. Whether you are dealing with their negativity or you are being inspired by them, their presence will help to shape who you are and what you think about. You could be reacting to them or worrying about them.

As you see their life unfold - their choices, their mistakes, their struggles and their victories, it opens you up to possibilities for your own life.

Their opinions will have an affect on you, positively or negatively. Sometimes their influence will challenge you to grow and change, and other times it will reassure you that you are doing just fine.

The people whose lives touch yours on a regular basis will have a strong influence on the way you live and how you grow.

Lighten Up!

Some people in our lives are like black holes, sucking the energy from us. They have no positive words, no listening ears, and offer nothing to support us. We are discouraged and frustrated whenever we spend time with them. They are not a good influence on us and we know it. We let them be our excuse to be lazy or gossipy. We know that we are not at our best when we spend time with them. These people are toxic to us and at some point we need to make a choice, a difficult choice.

It is difficult to get perspective on the point when a relationship has become toxic to you and it is time to step away from it. The fourth agreement can help you gain perspective.

If we strive to lighten up and take nothing personally we can get true perspective. Apply this agreement to all your relationships, including the energy sucking ones, it will help you see which relationships are truly toxic and which ones are there to help you grow.

Use the process below to help you gain clarity.

- Take a step back from the actions and words of your family members and friends. Objectively assess their effect on you. If you are feeling wounded or angry, first ask yourself if you are taking something personally that really is not about you. Do they have an issue that is part of their own drama and is not your drama? If it is affecting you adversely, can you let it go? Can you separate your reaction from their action? Can you lighten up about it?

- After taking a hard look at the situation and its effect on you, you must decide if this person is someone who you want to spend time with or not. Some relationships are temporary and we outgrow their purpose in our life. Give yourself permission to make the choice to release a friendship that is toxic for you.

- Family members can be the most toxic of all, but it might not be possible to release a family connection. Always remember to apply the agreement to take nothing personally with your family members as much as you possibly can. Remind yourself to lighten up and laugh at it all because there's a lot of "stuff" there.

If a family member is one of your toxic relationships, then minimize your interaction with them until something changes; either in you, in them, or in your circumstances.

Your "Social" Community

Choose the community that you associate with carefully; the group culture will greatly affect you. Nowadays, community is so much more that the town you live in.

Communities are any group environments that surround you. They are the social networks you choose, the clubs you belong to, the yoga studio where you attend classes, your co worker group, and the company you keep online. Yes, your Facebook, Pinterest, Google plus, Instagram and Twitter networks are all part of your social community.

The conversations, opinions, videos and links found online have an influence on you - so choose wisely where you invest your time. Before you click and randomly become a passive viewer of someone else's agenda, think about whether or not this post, this event or this conversation is worth your time and will it serve to enriched you in any way, shape or form. Do you want this influence or would it be better to pick up that fabulous book your yoga teacher told you about?

Be picky about your community - online and off.

To support Dan's efforts to bring music and joy back into the lives of people suffering with dementia and Alzheimer's, click here **www.CatherineMazurYoga.com/aliveinside**

PART FIVE

THE SPIRIT

*"You are not a drop in the ocean,
You are the entire ocean in a drop."*

- Rumi

Be!

Chapter Thirty Two
The Royal Path

"Every blade of grass has its angel that bends over it and whispers, 'Grow, grow.'"

- The Talmud

We live in challenging times. It's not unusual for people to feel overwhelmed, stressed out, worried or anxious. In fact, for many this seems to be the norm. When you ask a friend how his or her life is going you usually hear, "I'm busy" and "Life is moving so fast!" Sometimes we just want to stop the world and get off to take a breath.

The path of Raja yoga offers you relief. Often called the royal road, Raja yoga is a comprehensive path to turn our mental and physical energy into spiritual energy. The chief practice of Raja yoga is meditation which teaches you to become aware of your own state of mind. It is an ancient, time tested strategy to calm your nervous system and connect you to your deep inner reservoir of peace. This is an invaluable tool for healing and stress reduction.

In this section you will learn simple meditation techniques to rewire your brain and reduce stress, an easy plan for creating your own daily meditation practice and the science behind meditation and how it changes your brain.

Eight Royal Limbs

The royal path also includes all the methods we have discussed in the eight limbs of Patanjali's yoga which help us to control our body, energy, senses and mind in order to experience our true essence, which is spirit.

In review, the eight limbs of ashtanga yoga are:

YAMAS, The five moral restraints of nonviolence, truthfulness, nonstealing, moderation, and nonhoarding

NIYAMAS, The five observances of purity, contentment, zeal, self-study, and devotion to a higher power

ASANA, The postures, or the physical practice

PRANAYAMA, Mindful breathing

PRATYAHARA, Turning inward

DHARANA, Concentration

DHYANA, Meditation

SAMADHI, Union of the self with the object of meditation, blissful full awareness

Spiritual Beings On A Human Journey

On our earthly journey some of us enjoy exploring the limits of our physical ability, climbing mountains, running marathons, or doing yoga in 108 degree heated studios.

Why do we do it? For the challenge and fun of it! It makes us feel alive to test the limits of our physicality, and it gives us an emotional charge.

Another reason we seek to overcome the limitations of our bodies is our attempt to control life, which often feels out of control. We have limited power over life and the twists that fate hands us. We know our physical body will die, but have no idea how or when.

Change is inevitable and usually comes out of the blue, throwing us off balance. In working with extreme physical challenge, we feel like we've mastered the body and in doing so we feel as though we are in control.

Yogi masters take on the challenge of overcoming physical limitations by learning to control their body temperature and heart rate. These masters of Raja yoga aren't just trying to transcend challenges of life, instead their intent is to connect to their real essence; the essence that is spirit and unchanging.

Most of us don't devote our life to transcending our physicality as these master yogis do, but all of us are faced with challenges to overcome. We can apply the principles of yoga to help us navigate successfully through life's challenges.

Your Inner Roommate

How much of your life experience is physical? How much is spiritual? Emotional? Where do you have your greatest challenges and problems? Consider this - when a life problem is disturbing you, what part of you is being disturbed?

In his exceptional book *The Untethered Soul: The Journey Beyond Yourself*, Michael Singer refers to this disturbed part as your inner roommate. This roommate is always present with a reaction, melodrama or commentary. This roommate drives us crazy with incessant thoughts of worry, self doubt and criticism. It is the voice inside our head that is constantly jabbering away. When we try to quiet our minds or meditate, it is this part of us that will not be still.

But why should it be? Just as the function of the heart is to beat and pump blood and the lungs to breathe, the function of our human brain is to think. The brain is a thought producer, offering up thought after thought after thought. Anyone who has attempted to meditate is very familiar with the sensation of setting out to have no thoughts and be exasperated within the first sixty seconds by the tenacity of the brain to remain active.

To see this clearly and without a doubt, put the book aside and close your eyes. Tell yourself that for one minute you will have no thoughts. Set an alarm. Then watch and wait. Listen for the first whisper or half sentence to arise. Perhaps it will be more like a wisp of an idea or impulse. Try it now. Experience your brain creating thought on its own when you have determined to have no thought. It is close to impossible because we are in human bodies with human brains.

So then - who is it that determines to have no thought and then notices when thoughts arise on their own? When an emotion arises, or you have a thought that you don't want to have, take a step back and ask, "Who sees all this? Who notices?"

Asking yourself this question will cause you to look inside and see that there is an observer part of you that is noticing. The ability to notice our thoughts is essential to personal transformation. Once you can see that there is an observer part of you, you can ask yourself, "Who is it that sees?"

Then the truth begins to reveal itself that we are something else, something other than just human bodies and brains. There is a human self and another Self. The great sages and spiritual masters throughout the ages have taught that we are not humans on a spiritual journey, but rather we are spiritual beings on a human journey.

Discover the two aspects of spiritual practice,
the four aims of life and the five afflictions at
www.CatherineMazurYoga.com/rajayoga

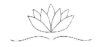

Chapter Thirty Three
What Is Meditation?

"...the point is to live everything.
Live the questions now. Perhaps then,
someday far in the future, you will gradually,
without even noticing it,
live your way into the answer."
- Rainer Maria Rilke, *Letters to a Young Poet*

*J*osh and Leah had been asking for a dog for a long time. We decided to surprise them with a golden retriever puppy for Hanukkah one year, and planned to hide her under our Christmas tree, aka our Hanukkah bush, so named because our household was a mixture of traditions and faiths which we simultaneously embraced and questioned.

We did a lot of searching for the perfect puppy that autumn; just as through the years we had done a lot of searching for the perfect spiritual path.

At that point, we were combining the traditions from both of our upbringings, but with a focus on Judaism. We had come to the realization that for us our prior religious labels were more of an identity than a set of beliefs. Because we loved the traditions from both the Christian and Jewish faiths we were raised with we celebrated both.

Over the first seven nights of Hanukkah, the kids opened one small gift each night, as was our tradition. On the eighth day, just before sundown, I picked up the puppy and put her under the tree, uh, the bush, closing the double louvered doors to the family room.

When the kids came downstairs to open their last gift, usually the biggest gift, they each received another small package. Leah's gift contained a collar and Josh unwrapped a leash. Their puzzled looks melted into big smiles as the puppy broke through the family room doors, impatient and unruly.

It was a really special holiday that year.

Their initial excitement and love for Ellie, as we named her, carried them through the challenges of training a new puppy - the whimpering at night, the peeing on the floor, and chewing of shoes.

They took on partial responsibility for training her which took some work and discipline and they learned that their beliefs about having a dog was different than the reality of having one.

It wasn't very long before the messes on the floor stopped and we could leave our shoes out without being chewed. During that time, they learned many valuable lessons, not only the work and value of discipline in raising a puppy, but also the importance of examining one's beliefs.

Ellie isn't with us anymore, but she changed us all forever. Josh and Leah have grown to be seekers themselves, examining their own lives with open hearts and minds. They learned that discipline has a very special reward, especially when applied to their own life journey with patience and understanding.

Training The Puppy

We are taught how to move and how to behave, but we are never taught how to be still and examine what is within. We were never trained to discipline ourselves to explore our inner self and understand our mind.

Our brain is the most unique and fabulous tool we have. It is the only one we have. As with any valuable and cherished possession, we need to care for it, keeping it trained and sharp, and rest it from time to time to keep it in prime condition.

With this tool, everything can be accomplished, including enlightenment, which is the objective of Raja yoga.

Meditation is the technique used in Raja yoga for training the mind to see itself. In it we are also training the brain to focus and rest.

As you learn to meditate, your mind needs the same kind of love, attention, and care you would show your toddler or a new puppy. Its first attempts to stop its wild ramblings and to focus on one simple thing will likely bring up resistance. Even though you decide to discipline and quiet your thoughts and even though your mind may try very hard to do as you ask, it stills wander off, since that's what it's always done. It has never been trained.

What Meditation Is Not

Many people tell me that they meditate every morning as they are laying in bed, waking up. While this is a useful practice, it is not the practice of meditation. Without a focused practice in place, this morning thought time is just thinking, day dreaming, fantasizing, or "vegging out."

On the other end of the spectrum, meditation is not a trance state in which the meditator loses touch with themselves and ordinary reality. It is not hypnosis or autosuggestion.

What Is Meditation?

Meditation is a simple technique of learning to pay attention to all the various levels of yourself. You simply observe and let the mind become quiet and calm.

It's a process in which we ask the mind to let go of its tendencies to think, analyze, remember, solve problems, and focus on the events of the past or on the expectations of the future. We help the mind to slow down its rapid series of thoughts and feelings and replace that mental activity with an inner awareness and attention.

By helping the mind to slow down, we are actually changing the pattern of our brain waves which produces a state of mind that is clear, relaxed and focused within, even if your inner state is anything but clear and relaxed.

We do this by employing various techniques to keep our brain focused and resting on one subject. Of the many techniques you can choose from, they all accomplish the same basic things which are:

- Training the brain
- Resting the brain
- Increasing awareness

Using your chosen technique, you learn to rest your mind and shift into a totally different state of consciousness than your normal waking state. This state of focused attention will actually change the pattern of your brain waves.

The basic intent is that you only want to keep in mind your meditation subject, whatever it is. Begin by simply observing and allowing your mind to become quiet and calm, exploring and experiencing deeper levels of your being. Easier said than done.

As you become more and more skilled at it, you will start to use the same faculty in your daily life to help you drop those thoughts that are unhelpful and become a master of your own thoughts, learning to choose the thoughts you want to entertain and release those you don't.

Ancient But Still Vibrant

Meditation has been around for a long, long time. All of the major religions have incorporated various forms of meditation, particularly in the mystical branches.

Ancient wall art dating back to 5000 BC depicts people sitting in the traditional meditation posture. There are descriptions of meditative techniques written about in the Indian dating back about 3000 years ago.

From the earliest civilizations it spread with the growth of humanity. Meditation is practiced in cultures and religions all over the world. But you don't have to follow any religious tradition to get the benefits of meditation. There are many, many types and techniques you can use to bring you into a meditative state. It is not the technique that is the meditation, meditation is the state of mind that the technique helps us to achieve.

Maybe you have experienced this meditative state in nature, surrounded by the magnificence of the mountains or ocean. All thinking stops and a deep presence and peace takes over. The Native Americans practiced this type of meditation by communing with nature.

The eastern Indian form of meditation was introduced to the United States in the early 20th century and popularized in the 1960s through the teachings of Maharishi Mahesh Yogi teaching Transcendental Meditation.

Now, over ten million American adults say they practice some form of meditation regularly including Oprah, Sting, and Ellen Degeneres. It is the key to unlocking your greatest potential and will give you something that nothing else can.

It introduces you to yourself on all levels.

Layers Of Awareness

The biggest misconception I encounter with my students is that meditation is somehow "stopping your thoughts." It is more accurate to say that meditation is sitting and sifting through the layers of your thoughts until there is a settling.

Even when you are sitting quietly there is a lot going on in your head.

First, there is the current train of thought that you are absorbed in. Put that aside. Not as easy as it sounds. Once you break free from the hold of those thoughts, like the clouds parting, there is another, deeper layer beneath it.

What's there? What lies below the surface thoughts? Another layer of thought, mood, agitation or preoccupation. Chances are, there is a theme to your thoughts. There is a constant dialogue that you default to day after day. Like a song on repeat, an endless loop ....that problem, those worries, your hurts or fears about the events in your life play over and over in the background. Every time you sit, this is what rises from the depths of you.

But wait - there is something else there. Awareness at another level. It might be the sound of the rain on the skylight or a distant bark of a dog that you become aware of when you begin to quiet your mind. Your brain registers the sound of the rain, just as it can hear the click of the computer keys in the adjoining room, but your mind has blocked them from your awareness while you are locked in worry. Releasing obsessive thinking allows you to tap into life as it unfolds. The rain, the present moment.

But as you listen more closely, even these fade to the background because there is an inner soundtrack. It could be the song you've been listening to earlier, still repeating in your head. Where is that music, lyrics, melody coming from? What is causing it to play over and over again of its own accord? This phenomenon causes you to be aware of another level of brain function occurring without your conscious attention to it. Amazing. What else lies at the depths of you?

If you shift your attention to your body you will notice the feeling of the clothes against your skin and the slight pressure of your feet on the floor. These are sensations you normally ignore - unless they become bothersome and they complain loudly enough to get your attention. Your hands on the chair, the temperature of the air, the fullness in your belly. Layers of awareness.

When you decide to get still and focus on what is going on in your mind with the intention of peeling away the layers, you begin meditation.

To meditate is to release the obsessive thoughts that normally occupy us. This is a very helpful practice because it gives us some reprieve from fears and concerns. Meditation is not the cession of thought, rather it is the process of dropping below your habitual worries, putting them to the side for a time while you focus on the immediate sensations of being alive. Relaxing and enjoying your senses to the extent that you can hear the background music playing soundlessly in your head.

Sometimes, if you sit long enough, you peel away the surface layers of awareness and get down to a layer that feels settled. You feel still. You've drifted down through the deep waters of your experience like sinking to the floor of a deep pond and resting there, peaceful, blissful. Most days the waters get stirred up quickly again and you don't rest in that stillness for long. The waves of thought and shifting currents of your experience wash over your stillness and you drift off again into the choppy waters of concern and preoccupation.

And that's okay. This is meditation. It is simply taking regular time to change the layers of your awareness experience and check the condition of the daily current of your thoughts. As you release layer after layer you are introduced to yourself in a way you haven't known before.

To begin your journey of meditation, go to **www.CatherineMazurYoga.com/meditations** for a basic meditation to get you started on your journey to awareness.

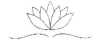

Chapter Thirty Four

The Benefits
of Meditation

*"You should sit in meditation for twenty minutes every day -
unless you're too busy - then you should sit for an hour."*

- Old Zen adage

*I*t was a muggy August day in Wisconsin, and the cousins were
together at the cabin with Mema and Bepa.

The cousins, ages three to eleven, had been in and out of the lake
all morning with squirt gun wars and now were busily building castles
on the beach. At noon, their grandmother called them in for lunch.

The macaroni was a big hit, but the apple juice was the natural,
unfiltered kind and they were sure there was something wrong with
it. They looked at the cloudy liquid in their glasses and said "YUCK."
Leaving juice glasses full, they returned outside to catch frogs.

In the afternoon heat, it didn't take long for the happy shouts to
turn into bickering voices and Mema could see it was nap time.

"What happened to those sweet kids from this morning? Come
inside and settle down." Strategically, she convinced them to watch a
movie and in 15 minutes most of them were asleep in front of the tv.

They woke happy and thirsty - all quarrels forgotten. Seeing that their juice glasses were filled with clear new juice, they gulped it down.

When Bepa returned from fishing, the kids excitedly told him about the squirt gun fight, the frog hunt and the yucky juice that they wouldn't drink until Mema gave them new juice.

"What new juice?" Mema said. "It is the very same juice from lunch. Just like you, it rested and changed. All the stuff that made it seem yucky settled down and it became clear."

It was their first lesson in meditation.

Just like that unfiltered apple juice, everyday stresses and concerns make us cloudy. As we sit in meditation, things begin to get clearer. The longer the glass sits on the counter, the clearer it gets. The longer we sit in meditation, the greater benefit we derive. Worries lose their importance and we connect to what really matters for us, leaving delicious clarity.

What is it about just sitting still that is so effective? How can sitting make these changes? Try it and see.

Meditation Is For Busy People

If just thinking about meditation makes you anxious, take a step back, look at the following definition and benefits and then reconsider.

Think of your meditation time as if you are creating clarity.

"Stillness is not about focusing on nothingness; it's about creating a clearing. It's opening up an emotionally clutter-free space and allowing ourselves to feel and think and dream and question."

- Brene Brown, *The Gifts of Imperfection*

If you have a busy, full life and are looking for some relief from its everyday stresses, meditation is for you. If you feel anxious, worried, or overwhelmed and long to rediscover the place of deep abiding peace inside yourself, meditation is for you.

The Research

Research studies show that meditation lowers stress levels, improves focus and concentration, and increases levels of happiness and well-being. In his book *Buddha's Brain, The Practical Neuroscience of Happiness, Love & Wisdom*, author Rick Hanson, Ph.D cites a number of studies which document the benefits of regular meditation. They include:

- Increases gray matter in certain areas of the brain
- Reduces cortical thinning due to aging
- Improves compassion and empathy
- Lifts the mood
- Decreases stress-related cortisol
- Strengthens the immune system
- Helps cardiovascular disease, asthma, type II diabetes, PMS and chronic pain
- Calms the nervous system
- Helps psychological conditions including insomnia, anxiety, and eating disorders
- Improves focus and concentration
- Deepens connection to inner resources
- Stabilizes emotions
- Provides access to deeper levels of creativity
- Increases awareness
- Restructures and strengthens neural pathways

What You Will Learn

To meditate, you'll need to learn how to:

- Relax your body
- Sit in a comfortable, steady position
- Make your breathing serene
- Witness the thoughts arising and traveling through your mind

Ultimately, you will learn to:

- Inspect the quality of thoughts and learn to promote or strengthen those which are positive and helpful in your growth
- Not allow yourself to become disturbed in any situation, whether you judge it to be either bad or good.

Simple Not Easy

Sounds simple, right? To get all those great benefits it takes some work.

It requires focus and discipline as we are teaching and training our brains. It is the same principle we employ when training our body. An untrained mind is like a wavering, fluctuating mass that runs from one subject to the next and finds it very difficult to stay in one spot. It is as unruly as an untrained puppy, and ultimately as unhealthy as an undisciplined body.

The mind has to be pushed to stay in one spot. It is like doing push ups or weight lifting. These are simple exercises - but certainly not easy! You will need to work hard to train your brain in the same way you would work to train your body.

Think of it as developing muscles in your mind. Strength can only come from exercising the mind to do exactly what one want it to do. We begin this training by teaching it to stand still in one place when you want it to stand still.

Just sit with it, like your puppy learning to stay, acknowledging how well it's doing. Notice when it goes astray and just bring it gently back to the task at hand. Don't expect it to get the hang of this new technique in just a sitting or two — but know that if you stay with it, your mind will become more and more able to stay focused and do as you ask.

The Force Behind Creation

The mind is not only the most valuable tool you have, but also the most powerful tool in all creation. Learning to focus creates a laser like energy that becomes the force behind creation. The continued focused attention you learn in meditation will spill over into other areas of your life. As you become aware of your patterns of thought and choose to focus continually on what you want your life to feel like, the law of attraction begins to magnetize it to you.

But don't take my word for it. Try it yourself and see.

There are many techniques to learn this focus and many types of meditation practice. Basically, during meditation we learn to drop from the mind what we don't want to keep and keep it single pointedly focused on the subject of our meditation.

As you become master of your own thoughts and learn to think what you want, you become an enlightened one, the master of your thoughts, feelings and your destiny.

The Dual Structure Of The Brain

The wisdom traditions of the world teach that the origin of the universe was one energy of reality (which is now known in scientific circles as the unified field theory) that polarized itself at the moment of creation into apparent dualities - good and evil, light and dark, male and female.

Interestingly enough, this duality, or opposition is also reflected in the structure of the human brain. The brain is divided into right and left hemispheres and in virtually all people, the two hemispheres are unbalanced, a state called brain lateralization. Because the brain filters and interprets reality in a split brained way, we tend to see things as separate and opposed, rather than as connected, unified. It predisposes us to see ourselves as separate from, and often in opposition to the rest of the world which creates feelings of stress, fear, anxiety and isolation.

In traditional meditation, the meditator seeks to eliminate the effects of brain lateralization through some form of focusing, such as repeating a mantra, keeping the attention on the flow of the breath, or some other focusing technique. As the meditator focuses, they move from a beta wave state, typical of normal waking consciousness, into a slower, more relaxed alpha brain wave state. Over time this relaxed meditative brainwave state leads to an increase in communication between the two sides of the brain and a less stressed state of mind. The brain changes and gradually new neural connections are made between the two brain hemispheres - in other words, the brain balances.

Binaural brain training is a meditative technique that is very effective in aiding the brain to create the beta brainwave state and thus balance the two sides of the brain. There are many programs that use brainwave entrainment and the binaural technology so help the meditator in his inner journey of awareness. In the following chapters will will explore a number of meditation techniques. Whichever you choose, you can also greatly benefit from a binaural approach to balancing your brain.

For more about how binaural brain training works and a link to an effective binaural program that can help you with meditation and create profound results, visit
www.CatherineMazurYoga.com/holosync

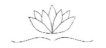

Chapter Thirty Five

How To Meditate

"The practice of meditation does not involve discontinuing one's relationship with oneself and looking for a better person. The practice of meditation is a way of continuing one's confusion, chaos, aggression, and passion - but working with it, seeing it from the enlightened point of view."

- Chogyam Trungpa

Uniquely Yours

If I had to tell you only one thing about meditation, it would be this: Meditation is your personal experiment, performed in the laboratory of your own mind and body. Your practice will be inspired by teachers. Yet, in the end, the form your practice takes is uniquely yours.

Finding Your Core Practice

Just as there are different paths one could take to climb a mountain, there are a variety of seemingly different meditation techniques. Yet all have the same goal - achieving a state of inner concentration, greater awareness, calmness, and serenity.

Look over the suggested practices and techniques in these two chapters and choose one you would like to start off with. Commit to that technique for a month. Remember though, the technique is NOT the meditation. The technique is a vehicle to lead you into the experience of meditation which is your unique experience.

A Basic Breath Meditation

1) Begin gently - be kind to yourself and don't expect too much

2) Get very comfortable, sitting upright and supported

3) Relax your body

4) Notice and follow your breath, focusing on each inhale and exhale

5) Let go and be patient

Let go of any negative thoughts that arise and instead close your eyes and feel your breath. It requires some precision to be right there with your breath. Be fully present with whatever is going on. You might be aware of outside sounds or sensations but as these distractions start to capture your attention, simply acknowledge them and them go. Simply sit right there, aware of your breath.

Poet and Zen master Thich Nhat Hanh says, "Watching and letting go: watching your breath and letting go of everything else."

WHAT YOU CAN EXPECT TO EXPERIENCE:

- Drowsiness
- Restlessness and a wild active mind
- Turbulent and unsettled feelings
- A sense of wellbeing or stillness
- Resistance to sitting

Remember, you are how you are, you are doing your best, so try to bring gentleness to the whole process. Avoid being critical of yourself and instead try to soften into the experience. Your meditation time should feel pleasurable, at least some of the time. You should get a certain enjoyment out of it, or you simply won't continue to do it.

Start with five or ten minutes and increase your meditation time one minute a day until you've reached a half-hour. It is very helpful to set a timer so that you are not preoccupied with the time. Give yourself completely to the experience, and when your timer chimes you will be refreshed.

A successful meditation practice requires balancing polarities: focus and letting go, structure and freedom. Your core technique is your jumping off point, it is the post you tie the puppy to. Stay with the technique that you have choosen for a month. Let it become comfortable and familiar, holding onto it loosely and at some points during your meditation, letting it go. An attitude of openness, expectation and awareness will guide you on your journey.

For guided meditations to take you deeper into your practice, visit **www.CatherineMazurYoga.com/meditation**

Chapter Thirty Six

Meditation Techniques To Help You

*"There are mornings when I get
caught up in an eddy of thought and
whirl there for the duration of my meditation.
Usually though whenever
I am able to apply one of these techniques with focus,
it takes me beneath
the choppy surface of my mind."*

- Danna Faulds,
Limitless, New Poems and Other Writings

Just Watch And Listen

When you sit in meditation, you watch your thoughts. You develop the ability to observe them as they arise. You develop the ability to allow them to dissipate without clinging to them or identifying with them. When you notice that you are following a train of thought, off on some tangent, you gently bring yourself back to your technique, releasing thought.

Don't be surprised if this watching and letting go of thoughts doesn't work all the time. Remind yourself to *stay* because, like an untrained puppy or a toddler, your brain will always try to dart away. Understand that usually during the first ten minutes the mind is calming down and quieting. Just keep sitting, watching and listening.

Keep in mind that you are not trying to change anything, and not trying to attain any state. The state you are in right now is enough. Consider that you are just witnessing the flow of mind: observing it without being disturbed or distracted.

As you listen, you become more conscious of the stories and emotions that your mind generates. Soon you can begin to distinguish between thoughts based on fear and thoughts based on truth.

Training your mind in meditation, you will begin to recognize your crazy stories, like "I'm not good enough" or "Nothing works out for me." As you learn to see clearly, you will realize this is the noise of your mind, and that you can accept or reject this noise.

Mantra

A really effective technique is to use a mantra in your meditation. Traditionally, mantras are sacred words given by a teacher to help the student awaken their divine essence. These mantras or sounds will have a specific meaning and vibration.

You can choose any sound or word that you want, such as "calm" when you inhale and "peace" when you exhale. The main point is to give your mind something to do that will act as an anchor to keep you focused.

There are also seed mantras which correspond to the seven main energy centers in the body. If you want to strengthen one of these chakras, you can use its mantra as you meditate.

If you are feeling anxious, fearful or long to be more grounded: Root Chakra - LAM

If you want to generate creativity and emotional stability: Sacral Chakra - VAM

If you want to foster personal power and change: Navel Chakra - RAM

If you want to become more joyful, loving and empathetic: Heart Chakra - YAM

If you have trouble speaking up and finding your voice: Throat Chakra - HAM

If you lack vision and want insight or knowledge: Brow Chakra - OM

If you want to connect to your higher self and detach from ego: Crown Chakra - OM

ENJOY IT

When you use a mantra, or any technique for meditation, there is a looseness about using the technique. You distribute your focus evenly between the technique, awareness and openness. You focus might look something like this:

25% is concentration

25% is openness

25% is awareness

25% is expectation

I hope this isn't sounding more complicated than it actually is. Perhaps this can be understood more fully with a metaphor. Buddhist meditation master Trungpa Rinpoche likens it to going to the movies and eating popcorn - a simple explanation from one who published six books, established three meditation centers and founded Naropa University in Boulder, Colorado. He explains that in meditation we maintain an inclusive focus of our entire experience, just as at the movies we have multiple focuses. At the movies 25 to 50 percent of your attention is on the screen, another 25 percent on the popcorn, and another 25 percent is on your companion. This all inclusive focus is what makes the entire experience pleasurable and ultimately develops enormous concentration.

Sensory Meditations

Using your senses as an anchor is another technique, especially for those new to focusing their mind. You can use any of the 5 senses to bring you into a focused state. Candle gazing is a common practice. Just light a candle at a comfortable eye gaze distance and become engrossed in the flickering flame. Remember to blink and feel free to set a timer.

Sound meditation is very relaxing and can be done listening to the sound of the wind, birds, classical music or chanting. Avoid music that has recognizable lyrics so that your thinking mind doesn't get caught up in the words.

Using prayer beads can be a touch meditation. Allowing a piece of chocolate to dissolve in your mouth mindfully is a taste meditation. Yummy, too!

No Excuse Meditation

However busy your life is, you can find time to begin a meditation practice. What is it worth to you to be happy? Is an hour to devote to meditation too much? What about the effort to think a positive thought and reject a negative?

You might not have 20 minutes to sit and meditate, but you can meditate for 1 minute twenty times a day.

Although I recommend 20-30 minutes daily, not everyone can begin and sustain that commitment. There is a way that even the most busy, unfocused person can meditate. I call it the No Excuse meditation, and you can find it with many other meditation tools on my website at
www.CatherineMazurYoga.com/noexcusemeditation

Chapter Thirty Seven
Lifestyle Practices

"For a long time it seemed to me that life
was about to begin - real life.
But there was always some obstacle in the way,
something to be gotten through first, then life would begin.
At last it dawned on me that these obstacles were my life.
And I saw that there is no way to happiness.
Happiness is the way."

\- Alfred D. Souza

PAUL'S STORY

I was diagnosed in 2006 with metastasized prostate cancer at 46 years old. It had traveled out of my prostate and into my bloodstream and bones. Very uncommon. The doctors gave me 2-5 years to live.

I didn't like that diagnosis, so I found a different doctor, a specialist, who said he could get me 10 years. And if he got me to 10 years, he could get me to 15.

I went through a year and half of everything but the kitchen sink. Ten weeks of radiation, five days a week, driving two hours each way for treatments, 18 weeks of chemotherapy in which I lost my hair and my strength, and then I got 4 weeks off to rebuild my body a bit.

During this treatment time, I was also on a hormone deprivation drug to treat the cancer. I would be on the drug for a while and then off for a "holiday" to rebuild myself up, which I needed because the treatments were wasting away my muscles and bones.

My core was jello. I wasn't done doing the things I wanted to do, like surfing and living my life. I desperately wanted to rebuild between treatments. Build back and maintain.

As I was looking for something to rehab me back from what the drugs were doing to my body, I heard from other surfers that yoga on a regular basis enhanced their sport. I thought, what the heck, why not do it? A friend hooked me up with Catherine.

I didn't know what to expect; I didn't really know all the benefits yoga provided on and off treatment, so I was not as committed in the beginning. All I knew was that I was headed into treatment again and didn't feel good.

When treatments started up again, I expected the same - during treatment every day gets worse. But soon I realized that bottom wasn't as deep and my rebound was quicker. I was seeing results and I got hooked.

I realized that yoga was helping to make my treatment periods easier and muscle wasting not as bad. Yoga brought me to a place where I began to consider a healthier lifestyle and have a better life. I became aware of what I was doing to myself.

Catherine told me, "Make some small changes that are sustainable - don't try to be perfect, just make it doable. Find an easy way to get good nutrition into your body. Drink something green!"

The first green juice I drank was at a great local health food store with a juice bar, Cream of the Crop. That was the start, but the big change happened when my wife committed to changing our lifestyle at home. It required the whole household to change their lifestyle of eating to live, not living to eat.

My kids benefit by the way we eat; my daughter knows how to read labels, and they are both acutely aware of what's good for them. They are educated about what creates disease.

What I am doing is keeping me alive. My cancer markers are low and stable. My doctor is amazed. I'm treating the cancer naturally with yoga and diet. I stopped putting things in my body that the cancer wants and opened up to big changes to bolster my immune system.

We don't know how long this will last, but now I'm in my 9th year and I've had the longest holiday ever in my treatment! Even if I have to go back into treatment, my whole goal is to have the longest holidays possible so I can enjoy my life.

At 55, I am as good of a surfer as when I was 20. I paddle on the surfboard with the confidence I haven't had since I was a young guy. It's important to me to live life fully; take the keys out of my hand and I won't be able to drive the car anymore in my life. I feel like I have the keys.

When Paul started doing yoga, he wasn't looking to change his life. He came to yoga out of desperation because nothing else had worked. He had to do something to feel like he was taking the reins of his life, the keys to the car back. Over time, as he practiced faithfully, the energy of yoga began to shift his perspective. He opened to the healing power of his own body, learning to support it by choosing to avoid foods that fed the cancer and by eating to live.

Synthia was drawn to yoga without knowing that it would be the catalyst to heal her deepest wounds. Her meth addiction was a symptom of a pain that she didn't know how to process. Yoga met her exactly where she was and gently allowed her to access and release her childhood anger.

Val was completely unaware that seeking emotional relief and healing for her back through yoga would take her down her perfect path of becoming a yoga teacher. It was only in the process of going through the practice that brought her, as it brings all of us, to the next step.

Samadhi

We are all looking for happiness.

Samadhi is the end goal of yoga. It can be defined as ecstasy and the experience of bliss. Sounds like happiness to me.

But how does doing yoga get you there? As author and teacher Pema Chodron says, "Start where you are."

Sometimes the only thing you know for sure is that you are in pain and desperate for change. Starting from that place, the first step is to develop compassion for your own journey and begin to practice any form of yoga that draws you. The next step is to question your old story and begin to let it go.

Let It Go

*Let go of the ways you thought life
would unfold; the holding of plans
or dreams or expectations - Let it
all go. Save your strength to swim
with the tide. The choice to fight
what is here before you now will
only result in struggle, fear and
desperate attempts to flee from the
very energy you long for. Let go.
Let it all go and flow with the grace
that washes through your days whether
you receive it gently or with all your
quills raised to defend against invaders.
Take this on faith; the mind may never
find the explanations that it seeks, but*

you will move forward nonetheless.
Let go, and the wave's crest will carry
you to unknown shores, beyond your
wildest dreams or destinations. Let it
all go and find the place of rest and
peace, and certain transformation.

- Danna Faulds, from *Go In and In*

When I began my journey down the path of yoga, I had no idea where it would lead me. I didn't even know what I was looking for and I had no concept of being separated from my true essence. I only knew I wanted to be happy and feel good in my body and my life.

Through yoga I've developed a deep understanding of what is truly important to me. The ancient path of yoga turns out to be a path which is consistently relevant and eternally powerful. My body is strong and healthy, my mind grows clearer and more aware. My lifework is rewarding and contributes to the community. As I help others on their path to becoming happy and free, I am amazed by how similar we all are; in our struggles and in our joys.

When I took my first class in that cold gym, I would never have believed that I would one day be writing this book, touching thousands of people's lives and training people to become yoga teachers. As I continue to practice, the path of yoga opens up to a wide road with countless opportunities to explore.

Change - real change - comes from the inside out. It doesn't come from looking for external quick fixes. It comes from making a decision and then showing up day after day to do the practice.

As you decide to walk down the path of yoga, it will be the consistent showing up that will take you to your next step, whatever that may be.

The paths of knowledge, action, devotion, and meditation are laid out before each of us. No matter which path you choose for yourself, it will be a rewarding journey, I promise.

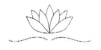

Resources

Here are a few resources that have been helpful for me and my clients. If you did not get a chance to explore, watch, or purchase these resources while reading the book, here is a list of all of the resources mentioned within the chapters of *Yoga Midlife Pain Relief Secrets.*

Abraham, Esther Hicks, and Jerry Hicks. *Ask and It Is Given: Learning to Manifest Your Desires*. Carlsbad, CA: Hay House, 2004. Print.

American Psychological Association. APA, Oct. 2008. Web. 30 June 2015. <http://www.apa.org/>.

Blake, Trevor. *Three Simple Steps: A Map to Success in Business and Life*. Dallas, TX: BenBella, 2012. Print.

Brown, C. Brene. *The Gifts of Imperfection: Let Go of Who You Think You're Supposed to Be and Embrace Who You Are*. Center City, MN: Hazelden, 2010. Print.

Chodron, Pema. *Start Where You Are: A Guide to Compassionate Living*. Boston: Shambhala, 1994. Print.

"DUJS Online." *DUJS Online*. Dartmouth College, 2015. Web. 30 June 2015. <http://dujs.dartmouth.edu/>.

Dyer, Wayne W. *The Power of Intention: Learning to Co-create Your World Your Way*. Carlsbad, CA: Hay House, 2004. Print.

Eden, Donna, David Feinstein, Brooks Garten, and Cindy Cohn. *Energy Medicine: Balancing Your Body's Energy for Optimal Health, Joy and Vitality*. London: Piatkus, 2008. Print.

Faulds, Donna. *Go in and In: Poems from the Heart of Yoga*. Greenville, VA: Peaceable Kingdom, 2002. Print.

Ford, Debbie. *The Right Questions: Ten Essential Questions to Guide You to an Extraordinary Life*. San Francisco: HarperSanFrancisco, 2003. Print.

Hanh, Nhat, and Mai Vo-Dinh. *The Miracle of Mindfulness: A Manual on Meditation*. Boston: Beacon, 1987. Print.

Hanson, Rick, and Richard Mendius. *Buddha's Brain: The Practical Neuroscience of Happiness, Love & Wisdom*. Oakland, CA: New Harbinger Publications, 2009. Print.

Harris, Bill. *Thresholds of the Mind, Your Personal Roadmap to Success, Happiness, and Contentment*. Beaverton, OR: Centerpointe 2007. Print.

Hawkins, David R. *Power vs. Force: The Hidden Determinants of Human Behavior*. Carlsbad, CA: Hay House, 2002. Print.

Kelley, Tim. *True Purpose: 12 Strategies for Discovering the Difference You Are Meant to Make*. Berkeley, CA: Transcendent Solutions, 2009. Print.

Kravitz, Judith. *Breathe Deep, Laugh Loudly: The Joy of Transformational Breathing*. West Hartford, CT: Free, 1999. Print.

McDougald, Alexandra. "Alive Inside." Alive Inside. Web. <http://www.lbhcf.org/programs-services/music/music-and-memory/>.

Rama. *Meditation and Its Practice*. Honsdale, PA: Himalayan International Institute of Yoga Science and Philosophy of the U.S.A., 1998. Print.

Roach, Michael, Christie McNally, and Patanjali. *The Essential Yoga Sutra: Ancient Wisdom for Your Yoga*. New York: Three Leaves, Doubleday, 2005. Print.

Robbins, Tony. "Ultimate Edge™ | Personal Development Program | Tony Robbins." <https://www.tonyrobbins.com/products/personal-growth-development/ultimate-edge/>.

Ruiz, Miguel. *The Four Agreements: A Practical Guide to Personal Freedom*. San Rafael, CA: Amber-Allen Pub., 1997. Print.

Siegel, Daniel J. *Mindsight: The New Science of Personal Transformation*. New York: Bantam, 2010. Print.

Singer, Michael A. *The Untethered Soul: The Journey beyond Yourself*. Oakland, CA: New Harbinger Publications, 2007. Print.

Trungpa, Chogyam, and Sherab Chodzin. *The Path Is the Goal: A Basic Handbook of Buddhist Meditation*. Boston: Shambhala, 1995. Print.

Vasey, Christopher. *The Acid-alkaline Diet for Optimum Health: Restore Your Health by Creating PH Balance in Your Diet*. Rochester, VT: Healing Arts, 2006. Print.

About the Author

Catherine Mazur is an acclaimed yoga and meditation instructor as well as a #1 International Best Selling Author and coach whose message is to use yoga to feel better. She is an innovator in personal development who has been featured on ABC, NBC, CBS and FOX News. Her unique philosophy bridges body, mind, and lifestyle practices to create meaningful, positive change in her life and the lives of her students.

Originally from Chicago, Catherine now lives with her family in sunny San Diego where she teaches, writes, and trains people to become yoga instructors. She embraces her yoga practice daily, and enjoys sharing her knowledge and insight with others.

You can find Catherine online at
www.CatherineMazurYoga.com